ANXIETY AND DEFENSIVE STRATEGIES IN CHILDHOOD AND ADOLESCENCE

ANXIETY AND DEFENSIVE STRATEGIES IN CHILDHOOD AND ADOLESCENCE

GUDMUND J. W. SMITH AND ANNA DANIELSSON

Psychological Issues
Monograph 52

INTERNATIONAL UNIVERSITIES PRESS, INC.
New York

Library of Congress Cataloging in Publication Data

Smith, Gudmund John Wilhelm, 1920–
    Anxiety and defensive strategies in childhood and adolescence.

    (Psychological issues ; monograph 52)
    Bibliography: p.
    Includes index.
    1. Anxiety in children. 2. Defense mechanisms (Psychology) 3. Child psychology. 4. Adolescent psychology. 5. Child psychopathology. 6. Adolescent psychopathology. I. Danielsson, Anna, 1949-   . III. Series. [DNLM: 1. Anxiety — In infancy and childhood. 2. Anxiety — In adolescence. 3. Defense mechanisms — In infancy and childhood. 4. Defense mechanisms — In adolescence.   W1 PS 572 monograph 52 / WS 350.6 S648a]
    BF723.A5S64   155.4'12   81-23633
    ISBN 0-8236-0389-X   AACR2

CONTENTS

ACKNOWLEDGMENTS

The project reported in this monograph was a joint enterprise from the beginning. Lena Sjöholm tested the pilot clinical group and half of the normal schoolchildren and helped in the first formulation of hypotheses; Maria Nordström tested the other half and co-authored the text on which Chapter 2 is based. Teachers at various levels of the Lund school system helped us to get normal subjects; the staff of the Children's Psychiatric Clinic provided us with clinical subjects and with valuable criteria. The late Professor Lennart Nilsson, head of the Psychiatric Clinic I at the Central Hospital in Lund, facilitated our work in various ways, above all by giving us work space. Many other people have assisted us in building our instruments, constructing our stimuli, processing our data, and typing our manuscripts. We wish to thank them all. Special grateful mention should be made of Sue Heinemann's competent editing of the manuscript.

Grateful acknowledgment is also made to the publishers to print revised versions of the following previously published material:

Gudmund Smith and Anna Danielsson, "Defensive Tendencies in Childhood and Adolescence as Defined by Process–Oriented Experiments," *Archives of Psychology,* 130:281–296 (1978).

Gudmund Smith and Anna Danielsson, "From Open Flight to Symbolic and Perceptual Tactics," *Scripta Minora, Lund,* 3:1–41 (1976–1977).

Gudmund Smith and Anna Danielsson, "Psychopathology in Childhood and Adolescence as Reflected in Projected Afterimage Serials," *Scandinavian Journal of Psychology,* 19:29–39 (1978).

Gudmund Smith and Maria Nordström, "Anxiety and Defense

Against Anxiety in Childhood and Adolescence," *Yearbook of the New Society of Letters at Lund,* pp. 67–102 (1975).

The research presented here was supported by a series of grants from the Swedish Council for Humanistic and Social Science Research.

INTRODUCTION

From 1972 to 1977 we conducted a series of studies on anxiety and defense against anxiety in children. Our work was based on percept-genetic techniques, as defined and described in a recent review (Smith and Westerlundh, 1980). These techniques provide an opportunity to analyze the successive stages in percept construction and reality adaptation. Given such a hierarchical perspective, an examination of the developmental aspects of children's percept genesis seemed inevitable. At the same time, our focus on anxiety and defensive strategies invited comparisons with psychoanalytic findings and speculations. Not only did our new, primarily objective methods allow us to take a fresh look at this old but controversial topic but, because our methods had previously been validated in various groups of adults, we could make systematic comparisons over a wide age range. Our results, it is hoped, will contribute both to dynamic theorizing about childhood and adolescence and to the introduction of new, objective assessment procedures.

We began our study with normal schoolchildren aged 7 to 15 years. Encouraged by the cooperative spirit of our young subjects, we decided to go as far down the age ladder as possible and include a group of 4- to 6-year-old preschool children. After these two studies of normal children, a comparison with children treated at a children's psychiatric clinic seemed natural and necessary in evaluating our findings. A pilot study of mal-

1

adjusted children guided our selection of children with anxiety as a key symptom.

DEFINITION OF ANXIETY

Our definition of anxiety closely follows psychoanalytic concepts, and our experimental techniques have been adapted to the structural-developmental view inherent in most dynamic theories of personality. By choosing a "mentalistic" approach to anxiety, we do not mean to deny the usefulness of alternative approaches, such as more neurophysiologically oriented ones. Anxiety is a broad and complicated subject, which cannot be tackled by any one set of tools or theoretical assumptions. It is important to emphasize, however, that the dynamic point of view need not — and should not — be nonbiological. Our interest in adaptive processes and the basic developmental perspective characterizing our research are implicitly biological in their focus on ontogenesis, even though we do not examine the specific physiological processes involved.

The psychoanalytic definition of anxiety, however, is ambiguous and old-fashioned in several respects. The lack of clarity about the concept of anxiety can be traced to Freud's *Inhibitions, Symptoms and Anxiety* (1926). Instead of disentangling the contradictions in Freud's text, we have relied on Schur's (1953, 1958) "redefinition" of anxiety:

> *Anxiety is a reaction to a traumatic situation, or to danger, present or anticipated. In this reaction we have to distinguish between the affect anxiety, which is an ego reaction, and the discharge phenomena, which are also id manifestations* [1958, pp. 218–219].

We shall explicate Schur's compact definition in adapting it to our theoretical model and empirical studies.

The reaction to an explicitly traumatic event is called *primary anxiety*. In quantitative terms, primary anxiety clusters at the high-intensity end of the spectrum, while reactions to anticipated danger are grouped at the low-intensity end. Anxiety, according to Schur, is associated with primitive discharge phenomena which the ego takes as positive evidence that a situation really spells danger. Such discharge phenomena as, for instance, flight or fight responses and vegetative symptoms are most openly displayed in primary anxiety.

Even if we did not accept the reaction to the trauma of birth as the prototype of primary anxiety, we would agree with Schur that primary anxiety, with its uncontrolled discharge, is most typical of very early stages in life. Phenomenologically similar kinds of reactions in older children or adults are generally referred to here as panic reactions or *paroxysmal anxiety*. The most prominent feature of paroxysmal anxiety is its sudden onset at maximal intensity. Paroxysmal anxiety is considered to be a regressive reaction.

Anxiety as a *reaction to present danger* implies, to paraphrase Schur, that some external object may initiate or end the traumatic situation; the danger is displaced to the condition determining that situation. In other words, diffuse discharge reactions are here superseded by less somatized and more focused reactions. Since the disappearance of the threatening object (or the anxiety-provoking absence of the object) may lead to an eventual cessation of the anxiety reaction, this kind of response seems to have many qualities in common with fright.

With *reactions to anticipated danger,* we reach a form of anxiety that is unthinkable without a representational world in Sandler and Rosenblatt's (1962) sense. The anxiety reaction is no longer bound to the appearance or disappearance of a real object but to the internalized representation of the object and various vicissitudes of that representation. We might phrase this: "I feel anxiety within myself." Quantitatively, reactions to anticipated danger are weaker than those described above; qualitatively, they are more colored by affect.

One interesting assumption in psychoanalytic theory, which is elaborated by Schur, is that in neurotic anxiety we are dealing with a temporary, partial ego regression, which may affect the evaluation of danger as well as the type of reaction to it. This ego regression may thus re-create a traumatic situation and cause a primitive form of discharge to reappear. While in the move from primary anxiety to internalized anxiety a desomatization usually can be observed, neurotic regression may instead lead to a resomatization.

In the chapters to follow we shall often use the term "parox-ysmal anxiety" as defined above. We also refer to "chronic anx-iety" to describe anxiety states of long duration and high intensi-ty that are not necessarily paroxysmal in form. Another com-mon term, "diffuse or free-floating anxiety," implies — to exploit Schur a last time — readiness for anxiety or a constant awareness of regressively evaluated danger. Here anxiety is based not so much on a present danger as on the anticipation of its imminent possibility.

DEFENSIVE REACTIONS TO ANXIETY

A basic assumption of psychoanalysis is that defensive reac-tions are triggered by anxiety or, to be more precise, by anxiety *signals* foreboding more violent discharge phenomena. Defenses may be directed against the painful affect itself or "against each link in the causal chain leading to the emergence of the painful affect" (Sjöbäck, 1973, p. 72). But anxiety is not the only painful affect in human experience. That depression, for instance, may trigger defensive reactions does not violate the hedonistic premise of psychoanalysis. It is still a question of avoiding unpleasure and promoting a safe and pleasurable homeostasis.

Yet many problems arise with the psychoanalytic postulation of an underlying pleasure principle. Critics have often pointed out that the organism itself may create disequilibrium in order, among other things, to further development. In our own study of normal creative adults, we have repeatedly encountered an obvious delight in the challenge of difficult and contradictory situations. These persons don't look for the "easy out." Instead, they choose the hard route because it will test and thus enhance their adaptive potential. They even seem to have a considerable tolerance for anxiety if it is likely to promote their creative aims.

In spite of all this, we shall assume that severe anxiety, or a signal of such anxiety, is likely to trigger various defensive countermeasures. In making this assumption, we accept the model of inner defense presented by Anna Freud (1936, 1970) and Otto Fenichel (1945), which has been further developed by ego psychologists. This model includes not only a hierarchy of defensive strategies built up around an ontogenetic sequence but also a hierarchy of anxiety manifestations. The association between type of defense and type of anxiety is, however, rather indirect in most clinical accounts. Here it will become an important focus of interest. We assume that anxiety reactions focused on external things call for a more direct, externally oriented type of defense than do internalized feelings of anxiety. Against really primitive anxiety, then, the only effective defense may be such phylogenetically ancient reactions as flight and freezing.

There will be ample opportunity to concretize these statements later. At this point we wish above all to emphasize the probable influence of a person's pattern of cognitive functioning on how the anxiety manifests itself and what kind of defensive strategy is used against it. The shift from a world of experience tightly bound to external objects to a world filled with internal representations implies a very drastic leap as far as cognitive maturity is concerned. We have made a special effort in our work to introduce such a cognitive perspective into the dynamic dimensions discussed so far. Our perspective is best represented by Piaget's developmental psychology. The particularly relevant principles of and stages in cognitive development will be elucidated in Chapter 1, when we discuss our use of Piaget's landscape test (Piaget and Inhelder, 1941, 1948).

Another important perspective for our studies originates in Heinz Werner's (1948, 1957) writings. Here we find a kind of double view of development: an ontogenetic and a microgenetic one. Both perspectives are characterized by the same steering principles. Following Werner, and ultimately Friedrich Sander (1928), we would say that the optimal cognitive level at which a person is capable of functioning (during a particular developmental period) is not arrived at once and for all but has to be reattained in each new encounter with the outside world. The adaptive process through which this mastery is achieved may eventually become more and more abbreviated and mechanized. When confronted with unexpected and trying circumstances, the person may once again adopt modes of experience and forms of behavior belonging to the distant, even very distant, past.

THE PERCEPT-GENETIC APPROACH

As we see it, the processes affecting a person's adaptation to the moment-to-moment requirements of the outside world are particularly useful as mirrors of the relation between the (experienced) self and the nonself. In our many research projects over the years at Lund University, we have paid particular attention to these processes, which we call *percept-genetic* (PG) processes, and we have constructed special tools to analyze how they unfold over a rather brief time span. The PG theory on which our method rests presumes (in accord with Heinz Werner and his predecessors) that everyday conscious perception is built up in a series of extremely rapid processes, which can be experimentally prolonged and thus made accessible to inspection by the psychologist. The roots of a perceptual process lie in a "general arousal" of previous personal experience, which is only vaguely tied to the stimulus; it primarily represents primitive aspects of self-other differentiation. From this subjective beginning, the PG process ideally leads to an unambiguous construction (perception) of reality, distinct from the perceiver. The stages preceding this concluding and objective C-phase are called P-phases.

Instead of describing in detail the developmental principles characterizing a PG process, we shall simply emphasize a few basic points (see Kragh and Smith, 1970, 1974; Smith and Kragh, 1975). One principle behind the microprocess of reality construction is *cumulation,* that is, a successive determination of form and content from phase to phase. In children, in particular, some of the contents of late phases cannot be referred to those of earlier ones. This acquisition of new experience is called *emergence.* If cumulation represents the principle of conservation, emergence represents advance, or growth, as it occurs at the forefront of the PG process. Another basic principle is *elimination.* There can be no stable C-phase if an increasing number of alternatives are not eliminated as irrelevant, marginal, or disruptive to the main course of development. We also need to take into account the fact that a number of early constructions, as well as the primitive modes of building and handling them, are relinquished during the PG process. *Dis-*

qualification is thus a fourth basic PG principle. It may be instructive to compare these PG principles, especially cumulation and disqualification, to certain assumptions about development in epigenetic theories: while incorporating previous phases, each new phase also represents a new level of organization and regulation (Gedo and Goldberg, 1973).

The PG process of reality construction can be studied only by *reconstruction* of its P-phases. Reconstruction must therefore be the main operating principle of any PG test. The tachistoscopic method of reconstruction involves presentation of the stimulus motif in such a way that it is only gradually correctly identified by the subject. The shorter the exposure time, the more aborted the PG process and the earlier the P-phase reported by the subject. By successively prolonging the exposure time, the experimenter can follow a series of P-phases up to the final C-phase. The meta-contrast technique (MCT) is a tachistoscopic method in which a "new" percept is generated within the frame of a percept established at the beginning of the experiment. By using incongruent or threatening picture motifs, the experimenter can specifically provoke anxiety and manifestations of defense against anxiety.

Another way to follow the process of reality construction is to confront subjects with an unusual perceptual phenomenon, to which they will adapt themselves over a series of repeated trials. In our investigations with children, we have employed an afterimage (AI) test shown to be sensitive to the presence of anxiety as well as to the subject's level of cognitive maturity. The subject is asked to report on the visual afterimage of a schematic face: to measure its size at a projection distance longer than the fixation distance, estimate its intensity, identify its color, and describe its general appearance. AI production is repeated several times, and the series of AI measures presumably reflects a process of perceptual adaptation.

One important characteristic of the PG tests is the way in which they illuminate the difference between the C-phase and the very early P-phases. The latter only vaguely reflect the stimulus. They can be characterized as offering a rich mixture of subjective contents, often condensed in a dreamlike fashion and specifically related to early personal experiences. This contrast between the primitive P-phases and the reality-proximal C-phase is very much akin to the difference between primary and secondary processes in psychoanalytic theory. Moreover, since the C-phase represents the present level of reality adaptation, content eliminated well before the C-phase might be compared to what psychoanalysts call latent content, as opposed to submanifest or manifest content.

Psychoanalysis, however, is not the only psychological theory implied in our reference to an epigenetic view. PG methodology also allows us to examine cognitive developmental tenets, above all those from the Piaget and Werner traditions. The concept of disqualification, for instance, reflects our view of development as a functional hierarchy in which primitive levels are continually superseded by more advanced ones. Since we use one Piaget's (1947) techniques to measure the cognitive maturity of the children in our various studies, we are naturally inclined to borrow his description of the cognitive developmental hierarchy. Yet the PG model also allows us to define the concept of regression in the spirit of Werner (1948), implying a return to more primitive forms of activity or a dedifferentiation of the present level of functioning. In this regard, if the PG process is prevented from reaching its C-phase, discarded and more diffuse or syncretic functions at a P-phase level may again be decisive in determining the subject's adaptation to reality.

The affinities between psychoanalysis and the Piaget-Werner tradition have often been pointed out, especially by outsiders (Gardner, Jackson, and Messick, 1960). Yet they are rarely connected on an empirical level. In recent years, however, several psychoanalysts seem to have realized how useful Piagetian developmental ideas can be in highlighting and complementing dynamic concepts. Insightful comparisons have been offered by A. M. Sandler (1975) and Greenspan (1980). In any case, the two traditions combine naturally within the operational framework of the PG approach. Our first investigation, with normal schoolchildren, will clearly demonstrate that they supplement each other in important respects as far as children's defenses against anxiety are concerned. Anxiety manifestations and defensive strategies cannot go beyond the limits set by the child's cognitive maturity which, in its turn, may be halted and thwarted by the degree to which anxiety dominates the child's experience.

1

METHOD

Before describing the results of our experimental work with children, we shall explain in some detail the tests we chose to study anxiety and the strategies used to defend against it. As we noted in the Introduction, tachistoscopic techniques can be used to prolong and analyze the PG processes behind everyday perception of reality. Previous work with adults has shown the afterimage (AI) test and meta-contrast technique (MCT) to be useful measures of the effect of anxiety on reality construction (see Smith and Kragh, 1967; Smith, Johnson, Ljunghill-Andersson, and Almgren, 1970). In addition to these two tests, we used Piaget's landscape test to gauge the cognitive maturity of the child, as this too affects reality construction.

We shall begin with a description of the AI test, as the data from this test often served as a background for the interpretation of the MCT results, particularly along the dimension of anxiety.

Afterimage Test

In order to comprehend how AIs can be of value in personality description, we have to examine in some detail the place of the AI phenomenon in the individual's field of experience. That the subject is not entirely new is attested to by many publications from the early part of this century (Kroh, 1922; Jaensch et al; 1929, 1930; Vujić and Levi, 1939). Serial experiments with AIs began with an early twin study (Smith, 1949), continued in a monograph on *Aktualgenese* by Kragh (1955), and were resumed again, after more than a decade, in a study of anxiety (Smith and Kragh, 1967). The bulk of work on AIs and other visual aftereffects performed in Lund has been presented in a special monograph (Andersson, Nilsson, Ruuth, and Smith, 1972). Many of the most recent studies on AIs have used children as subjects.

In considering the developmental significance of AIs, it is useful to conceive of two poles to the person's experiential world: the self and the nonself (see Andersson, Johansson, Karlsson, and Ohlsson, 1972). This polarization of experience into what belongs to us and what belongs to an independent outside world undergoes a series of changes during development. Following Piaget (1923; Piaget and Inhelder, 1966), we may distinguish the first three important stages in the child's cognitive development from about 4 years of age:

1. An early preoperational stage, with fragmentary "internal representation" and a still rather diffuse differentiation between self and nonself.

2. A later stage, where thought becomes more separated from action, and the self is more clearly set off from the nonself, but internalized actions are still tied to perceptual rather than cognitive criteria; the overall perspective is thus egocentric, with the nonself dominated by the self.

3. The stage of concrete operations, where perceptual appearances no longer dominate thought processes and the egocentric perspective is replaced by a more relativistic one.

AIs have proved rewarding as PG tools above all because of their ambiguous position in the phenomenal world; they "present themselves" somewhere in the region between the self and the nonself poles of experience. Although an AI appears in the world surrounding the observer, it is not part of this world—it moves with the observer's eye movements; it does not in fact cover the objects against which it is projected; it disappears and then reappears. Through consecutive presentations of a stimulus that will induce an AI, it is possible to study how this ambiguity is eventually resolved by the subject. One obvious prerequisite for this kind of experiment is that the subject not be presented with the AI phenomenon beforehand or with any kind of AI theory.

At a developmental stage where the self and the nonself are still undifferentiated, we would not expect the child to produce any AIs at all. Such a young child cannot even understand what Piaget's landscape test, with its choice of perspectives, is all about (see the description below and also Chapters 3 and 5). These findings apply to children at the first stage of preoperational thinking. At the next stage children readily project AIs and can measure their size on a screen. Lacking an outside perspective on themselves, however, these children see the AIs as part of the external, physical world. Hence, in their reports, the AI is likely to retain the color of the initiating stimulus and to increase very little in size when the projection distance is lengthened (Ruuth and Smith, 1969; Ruuth and Andersson, 1971). Their AIs are also more sensitive to changes in the projection surface (Smith and Sjöholm, 1972). Not until the post-egocentric stage does the mature AI appear, the well-known negative image which changes in size with the projection distance.

AIs, however, should not be viewed only from a cognitive perspective. Since AIs are part of our experiential world, they may be emotionally colored. In other words, even the adult AI cannot be regarded merely as the mechanical result of certain conditions pertaining to the stimulus and projection surface. In persons suffering from manifest anxiety, for instance, we have found that AIs become dark, even frightening, or cover an increasing portion of the perceptual field (Smith and Kragh, 1967; Smith, Sjöholm, and Nielzén, 1976). It has also been demonstrated that when anxiety is curbed by depressive retardation, AIs are likely to gradually diminish and lose their darkness over the experimental series (Smith, Kragh, Eberhard, and Johnson, 1972). Alternatively, in compulsive subjects the dark color (indicating anxiety) may be blocked by certain subtle shifts in hue (from blue or blue-green to clearly green with a red stimulus), making it difficult for the AI to become oversaturated, achromatic, or black (Andersson, Fries, and Smith, 1970; Smith, Fries, Andersson, and Ried, 1971).

Because the experimenter uses the same stimulus in repetition and requires the subject to project a new image after each presentation, the AIs reflect an adaptive process. If enough trials are administered, such a serial AI experiment will allow for the optimal adaptation of each subject to the AI phenomenon. The early phases in the experiment can, then, be seen to reflect adaptive stages "left behind" by the individual, i.e., those which are no longer part of the person's everyday reality perception. The AI process thus reproduces the hierarchical stratification of the individual's experiential world. An AI serial initially characterized by very primitive images may well show mature images at later stages, but the early dominance of immature AIs may indicate a potential for regression if the adaptive task becomes difficult.

Diagnostic work utilizing AIs is based on the assumption that, eventually, the perceiver will conceive of the AIs not only as phenomena emanating from himself[1] but from a very limited part of himself, an isolated sense organ. The AI process, in this case, ends with an image reflecting the stimulus and projection situation in a predictable, "physicalistic" way. If, however, the perceiver (child or adult) is given a different theory about the "true" nature of AIs, this course may be disturbed. It is possible, by means of explaining the AI phenomenon in various ways, to produce childish AIs in adult subjects or AIs with a particular emotional coloring (Smith and Sjöholm, 1974a). Nevertheless, given the prevailing scientific world-view, the natural end-product of the AI process in adults is the kind of image described in most textbooks.

TEST PROCEDURE

The AI apparatus consisted of a semitransparent, ground Plexiglas screen (23.5 × 23.5 cm), movable along two horizontal bars. Two markers at the front of the screen could be moved independently of each other, by means of two levers. The subject pulled the levers toward himself to measure the width of the AI.

The stimulus was projected from behind the screen, and the subject viewed it through a tight-fitting eyepiece. The room was faintly illuminated (ca. 1.4 lux at the screen). The stimulus was a relatively intense (ca. 50 lux) red figure with straight sides and rounded contours at the top and bottom. It had two eyes and a down-turned mouth schematically drawn in black. The "sad" mouth was chosen because a previous study (Fries and Smith,

---

[1] Throughout this monograph we have adopted the generic use of the pronouns "he," "his," and "himself" to describe both male and female subjects. This choice has been made primarily to avoid the cumbersomeness of the "he/she" construction. The missing female pronoun should be kept in mind by the reader.

1970) had shown that with this stimulus we obtained more variation in our scoring dimensions than with a "neutral" or "happy" mouth. A black fixation point on the screen coincided with a nose. The width of the stimulus was 5.5 cm. The subject fixated on it for 20 seconds. The fixation distance was 39 cm and the projection distance 59 cm. The expected Emmert size of the AI was thus 8.3 cm. (The red color of the stimulus figure can be defined by the transmission values of the color filter [20% at wavelength 3800, close to 0% at 4500–5500, 50% at 6000, and 90% at more than 6500] and by the make of the projector lamp [Philips 6158 N/05, 100W, 230V].) In order to extinguish the AI, a diffuse red light was exposed for five seconds after each trial, if necessary.

Sixteen trials usually comprise a series for adult subjects because after this number of trials AIs do not change appreciably. Our subjects, particularly the younger children, could hardly be forced to endure such a long and trying session. Accordingly, the number of trials was cut to 10. The time required per trial was about 70 seconds.

The brightness of the AI is usually judged on a 10-point scale. To guide this intensity estimate, a light and a dark field are exposed on the screen before the red face is shown. These two fields serve as anchor points for the intensity scale; the light field represents 1 and the dark one, 10. However, subjects are also allowed to use one additional step (>10) if the AI seems "blacker" than the dark field. In our sample many children could not fully understand how to use such a rating system. They were therefore asked to give a cruder estimate (light-medium-dark) of AI brightness (with particular attention given to the dark end of the scale), along with their description of color and general appearance.[2]

Scoring Dimensions

The main scoring dimensions in the AI test are size, brightness, and color. Another characteristic of some interest is a subject's inability to produce an AI after more than two trials.

---

[2] Children suspected of color blindness were tested with the H-R-R Pseudoisochromatic Plates.

Reports of physiognomic AI characteristics (e.g., a smiling face, teeth in the mouth, a giraffe instead of a face) are also noteworthy.

Several AI characteristics have proved to be useful diagnostic signs in adults. Dark (intensity ratings of 10) and/or large (10.5 cm or more) AIs (other than at the beginning of the test series) are common in adults with manifest anxiety. Abrupt changes from normal-size AIs (8.3 cm) to size-constant ones (6.5 cm or less), or from negative to positive AIs, are found in schizophrenics and are interpreted as signs of regression. More permanently size-constant or positive AIs are typical of immature subjects. In depressive patients, the AI series is often characterized by continuously shrinking size or decreasing darkness, which could be seen as a reflection of depressive retardation. These and other characteristics of adult AIs are presented by Andersson, Nilsson, Ruuth, and Smith (1972), together with references to previous validation (and cross-validation) studies.

The scoring dimensions used in our experiments with children and adolescents will be detailed in the presentation of our data.

META-CONTRAST TECHNIQUE

The MCT dates back as far as 1952, when George S. Klein and the senior author were testing methods to operationally define tolerance for ambiguity. One such method involved the successive presentation of two schematic faces, one sad and one happy, in a tachistoscope. We asked how long the exposure time would need to be before the subject could identify both contrasting stimuli. The question was never answered because the pilot subjects did not behave as expected. If, at that time, we had checked the work on perceptual contrast by Werner (1940), Cheatam (1952), and others, we could have predicted that the first stimulus would be masked by the second one.

Other reactions were even more surprising. When a smiling face was presented before a neutral one, by which it was masked, some subjects added emotional coloring to the second face.

For instance, while pointing out the neutral expression of the mouth, some described the eyes as twinkling with suppressed mirth. This discovery of the subliminal effects of the masked stimulus in a meta-contrast design was the starting point for a long series of studies on subliminal perception (Smith and Henriksson, 1955; Klein, Spence, Holt, and Gourevitch, 1958; Smith, Spence, and Klein, 1959).

The MCT has also yielded results of diagnostic interest. Smith and Henriksson (1956), using pairs of incongruent stimuli, found that the subliminal effects were particularly dramatic in paranoid patients. The perceptual process triggered by the masked stimulus (A) did not lead to an independent perception of A (whether correct or incorrect), but only to reports of changes (often drastic ones) in the masking stimulus (B). In other words, the subject did not say: "There is something new coming into B," but rather: "B is different." The perception of A was thus merged with the process leading up to the conscious perception of B. This seemed to be an adaptive strategy analogous to the workings of the defense mechanism of projection, where a subject may refuse to admit, for example, his own aggressive impulses and instead perceive aggression in the behavior of other people. Similarly, it was found that persons who used isolation for defensive purposes also isolated the masked stimulus from their conscious percepts and reported no subliminal effects in the MCT situation.

Our personality-oriented work with the MCT has been influenced by the emphasis on cognitive style found in the early work of George S. Klein and his associates (Klein and Schlesinger, 1949; Holzman and Klein, 1954) and by an interest in PG processes initiated during the 1940s by a group of young psychologists at Lund University. The first influence, in particular, directed our attention to the formal attributes of adaptive strategies and motivated the choice of such incongruent pairs of stimuli as the car and room used in one of our MCT series. An interest in events over time, even microtime, then contributed to making the MCT an instrument for the analysis of how a new percept develops within the frame of a stabilized one. The stabilized percept was the masking stimulus (B), to which the subject had been adapted beforehand; the new perceptual process was initiated by the masked stimulus (A), presented to the subject in short time periods and thus only gradually allowing him to reach the final stage of correct identification. The advantage of viewing cognitive style as an event over time has also been demonstrated in studies of adaptation to color-word interference (Smith and Klein, 1953).

As we just noted, the data from the inquiry into the perceptual style of a person confronted with incongruent stimuli illuminated normal personality characteristics as well as pathological symptom formation. The parallel development of a test originally intended to screen airplane pilots—the Defense Mechanism Test, or DMT (Kragh, 1969)—inspired us to supplement the incongruent stimuli with pairs in which stimulus A_2 represented a threat and stimulus B_2 included a person against whom the threat could be said to be directed.

In pointing out this similarity between the MCT and the DMT, however, we should not overlook the considerable differences between them. In the DMT the experimenter uses one stimulus picture, in which the threat is placed in a peripheral position. The MCT employs two different stimuli. Here interest is centered not only on the development of A but also on how the subject's ordinary field of perception (his report of B) is influenced by the developing, new, incongruent or threatening percept. The difference between the MCT and the DMT as diagnostic instruments has been described by Palmquist (1974).

The choice of incongruent or threatening stimuli was motivated by a desire to induce a small amount of additional anxiety in our subjects and thus facilitate defensive operations. In order to learn how to read the subject's perceptual reports with an eye to defensive activity, an extensive validation program was started in the late fifties. The early results were reported in a manual (Smith, Johnson, Ljunghill-Andersson, and Almgren, 1970; see also Kragh and Smith, 1970), but the validation work is still going on. The initial emphasis was on adaptive and defensive characteristics in adults, particularly adult psychiatric patients. The focus of attention has now shifted to children, including both normal and clinical subjects. Although the interest in defensive formations remains, especially with regard to early precursors of adult strategies, the interest in anxiety per se has increased.

Tests like the MCT and DMT have much in common with conventional projective tests. Knowledgeable readers will probably detect that some scoring principles used in the Rorschach test appear in disguised form in the MCT. However, as pointed out by Kragh and Smith (1970), the process emphasis of the PG method sets it apart from these other tests. A PG test involves the reconstruction of a perceptual process which (1) usually occurs in microtime, unnoticed by the perceiver, and (2) grows out of an individualized functional context, but ideally leads to an "objective" percept, free from subjective coloring. The early reports in a PG test (P-phases) are most likely to be typical of primitive, ontogenetically "early" functional levels of the perceiver, while reports closer to the final recognition of the stimulus (the C-phase) are expected to reflect more directly the subject's present functional status. A differentiation between early (latent) and late (manifest) signs in a PG test may therefore be important, particularly with adult subjects.

Test Procedure

The MCT has been described in detail by Kragh and Smith (1970) and in the Swedish manual (Smith, Johnson, Ljunghill-Andersson, and Almgren, 1970). Figure 1.1 illustrates the procedure for the threat series. The test involves the tachistoscopic presentation of paired stimuli (A and B). In Series 1 stimulus A_1 (a car) is incongruent with stimulus B_1 (a living room), while in Series 2 stimulus A_2 (a threatening face) implies a danger to B_2 (a young person [most often seen as a boy] sitting at a table with a small window in the background, where the threatening face is projected). B is first presented at gradually prolonged exposure times. (Starting with 0.01 seconds, exposure steps are arranged in a geometric series with a quotient of $\sqrt{2}$.) When the subject has reported B correctly, the exposure time is reduced to a standard level (about 0.06 seconds). Presentations of B at this level constitute a control series which, unnoticed by the subject, continues into the main series, where A is exposed immediately before B. While the exposure time of B is kept constant, that of

MCT Stimuli

A_2 = A threatening face.

B_2 = A boy (girl) sitting at a table with an object (presumably a violin) in front of him (her) and a window on the left wall (where A_2 is eventually going to appear).

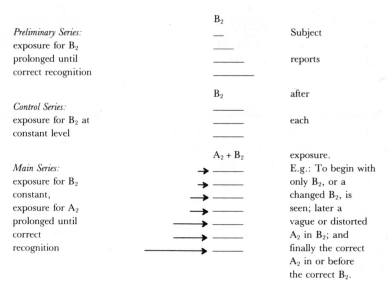

FIGURE 1.1

SCHEMATIC ILLUSTRATION OF THE THREAT SERIES IN THE MCT

A is gradually prolonged every second time until A + B have been correctly reported in three consecutive trials.[3]

Subjects are told to report everything they see on the projection screen for each trial. The instructions are: "We are going to show pictures on the screen. They will come in brief flashes. I will therefore say 'now' before each presentation. Look at the screen when I say 'now' and tell me afterward what you saw."

The following minor deviations in our studies from standard procedure should be noted: (1) While the schoolchildren sat at a distance of 1.6 m from the screen (the distance used with adults), the normal and the clinical preschool children sat about 50 cm closer to it. (2) Because all the preschool children could not endure protracted testing, they were generally given only

[3] For obvious reasons, retesting with a particular MCT program is not possible. A parallel version with one incongruent and one threat series has been constructed, which is to be given after the first one. It was not used in the studies reported here.

single presentations at each exposure level in the A + B section. (3) If necessary, a short pause was inserted between Series 1 and Series 2. (4) The experimenter not only recorded what the subjects reported but also *how* they behaved in the situation. (An exception to this last point was the study of normal school-children.)

Scoring Dimensions

The scoring dimensions will be detailed in our presentation of our data. Series 1 is mainly used for scoring developmental discontinuities and subliminal effects, and Series 2 for scoring anxiety and defensive structures. Both series belong together in a complete testing session.

Using as concrete and explicit descriptions of the dimensions as practically possible, we were able independently to arrive at very similar results when scoring the protocols. Minor divergences were settled in discussions. High interrater correlations have previously been reported by Almgren (1971).

The scoring was usually restricted to + (for certain presence) and – (for absence). In a few cases, (+) was used for doubtful presence; these instances are explicitly noted in the text. In order to differentiate between early and late signs, we also counted the number of exposures, beginning with the first A + B presentations and ending with the C-phase, i.e., the first exposure in the triad of correct recognitions (if any). Late signs were defined as those appearing in the last third of this exposure series and early signs as those appearing before.

Scoring of Anxiety

The first indicator of anxiety to be postulated was the subject's reporting dark or black forms (Smith, Johnson, Ljunghill-Andersson, and Almgren, 1970). A subject might describe black clouds in the window or particularly emphasize the darkness of the wall behind the "hero" (the young person in B_2). The correlation between this sign and symptoms of anxiety, however, was only moderate compared with, for example, the correlation between varieties of defensive isolation in the test and compulsive symptoms.

In a later work summarizing the scoring of anxiety in adults (Smith, Sjöholm, and Nielzén, 1976), an important qualification was added. The authors scored anxiety "not only when dark formations [appeared] but also when formations offering protection [from] the threat were impaired or disappeared" (p. 153). According to them, the more frequently the protective features had been reported before their breakdown, the more intense the resulting anxiety would be. Three levels of anxiety were then distinguished:

1. The B_2 picture as a whole disintegrates or is in some way damaged; the formation corresponding to A_2 becomes impaired or disappears after repeated reports of a stimulus-distant, inanimate object (a phobic formation) or a human face.

2. A phobic formation is reported once and then bcomes impaired or disappears; the window becomes grey or diffuse, rain-streaked, shadowed; dark areas become prominent; the whole atmosphere seems more forbidding or disquieting.

3. Relatively different reports show successive deterioration.

Subsequent validation work with a group of anxiety-ridden adults revealed that the signs at the highest level correlated better with symptoms of manifest anxiety than did the other signs. Among the severe signs were reports in which B had lost all meaningful content (zero-phases), or its components were perceived as broken or on the point of breaking (full of holes and cracks), or an independent, clearly defined image corresponding to A later completely disappeared. Signs scored in the latter part of the A + B series were found to be more valid than signs scored in earlier parts.

Scoring of Defensive Reactions

Defensive reactions in the MCT may manifest themselves in many different ways. As we shall see later, a child or very immature adolescent often simply denies what is presented on the projection screen. Previous work with adults has particularly emphasized defenses at the perceptual level, stressing that the threatening face in Series 2 is not recognized as such but may be changed to something more acceptable, omitted, hidden, or forgotten. The defensive tactics are numerous. In the manual

(Smith, Johnson, Ljunghill-Andersson, and Almgren, 1970), these signs are characterized as repressive, hysterical, compulsive, paranoid, etc. In addition to clear-cut defensive reactions, previous studies have also considered depressive and psychotic responses (the latter are mainly characterized by process discontinuities).

Since it would be difficult for the reader to keep a long and varied scoring catalogue in mind, we shall discuss the particular defenses in the light of our data. Here it may suffice to cite some of our basic sources from the validation work with adults: Kragh and Smith (1970); Å. Nilsson and Almgren (1970); Almgren (1971); I. K. Nilsson and Larsson (1972); Holley and Nilsson (1973); Hagberg (1973); Smith, Sjöholm, and Nielzén (1974, 1975, 1976); Magnusson, Nilsson, and Henriksson (1977). We also offer a few illustrative examples.

Series 2

Repression: The subject reports A_2 as a lifeless bust or a mask, instead of a live, threatening face. This kind of report is particularly common in primitive hysterics and, to use psychoanalytic terminology, could be interpreted as a decathecting of the threat.

Isolation: A_2 is seen as a harmless white spot, as curtains covering the window in B_2, etc. This "isolating" response is typical of compulsive subjects.

Both Series

Projection: Instead of reporting A as a new structure within B, the subject suppresses A and reports changes in B, e.g., persons in the living room in Series 1 but no car. Projective reactions are typical of paranoid subjects.

Discontinuity: The subject suddenly reports a chaos of lines or total darkness, for example, instead of B (or A + B). Such zero-phases usually indicate severe psychotic disturbances.

Like the signs of anxiety, the signs of defense and adaptive irregularities were more representative of manifest symptoms if they were scored in the latter part of the A + B series.

LANDSCAPE TEST

The landscape test (Piaget and Inhelder, 1941, 1948) was

used to measure the degree of egocentric thinking. In this test a model of a mountain with three (differently shaded) peaks is placed before the child, who has at his disposal four photos of the landscape, each taken from a different direction. A doll is then placed in these viewing positions, one after the other, starting with the child's own position. The child has to choose the photo that represents the doll's perspective.

A child dominated by egocentric thinking will prefer the photo showing his own perspective, but a pre-egocentric child will not know how to choose at all, even when the doll is located in his own place (Smedslund, 1967). This is the main reason why "own" perspective was included in our version of the landscape test (although it was not used with the normal schoolchildren). It should also be mentioned that the child was not told if his choice was correct. If the experimenter was uncertain whether the child had really tried to choose between the photos, the child was asked to try again in order to promote optimal performance.[4]

---

[4] Except for the normal schoolchildren, all children were handled by the same person.

PART ONE

NORMAL CHILDREN

2

INITIAL STUDY OF
NORMAL SCHOOLCHILDREN

A study of 72 normal subjects, ranging in age from 7 to 15 years, served as the background for subsequent studies of 4- to 6-year-old normal children (Chapter 3) and of children with symptoms of anxiety (Part Two). Although this initial study included a pilot group of clinical children, as well as a small "adult" group of 19-year-old military conscripts, many of our conclusions must remain rather hypothetical until the results of the subsequent studies have been reported. Only then will we be able to draw a complete picture of how anxiety and its vicissitudes are reflected in PG data and how defenses operate to counter this anxiety.

Several specific points of interest guided our study of anxiety and defense in normal schoolchildren. One such concern was to compare the characteristics of children just before or on the verge of puberty (our [11]12–13 age group) with those well into puberty (our 14- to 15-year-olds).[1] We also intended to search for precursors of typical adult defensive strategies, as well as to inquire into the role of cognitive maturity in the manifestations of anxiety and methods of defense. These special goals aside, the overall purpose of our first study (and of the subsequent ones included in this volume) was to illuminate how anxious children function and how they experience themselves in relation to the world around them. Given the developmental per-

---

[1] The decision to call the (11)12–13 age group "prepuberty" was based on the fact that these children were not yet sexually mature. The boys were still sopranos and only a few of the girls had started to menstruate. As Tanner (1971, p. 202) indicates, the age of menarche is somewhat later in Sweden than in Great Britain or the United States. The youngsters in this prepuberty group clearly differed from the 14- to 15-year-olds, who were definitely in the thrall of puberty and the problems of early adolescence.

TABLE 2.1
AGE AND COGNITIVE MATURITY GROUPS
OF NORMAL SCHOOLCHILDREN

Group	Landscape test	N	College-educated father
Age 7–8			
Immature	≥ 1 error	9	4
Mature	0 errors	7	3
Total		16	7
Age 9–10(11)			
Immature	≥ 2 errors (3)*	10 (2)	3
Mature	< 2 errors (< 3)	10 (2)	6
Total		20	9
Age (11)12–13	0 errors	17 (4)	7
Age 14–15	0 errors	19	8

*Figures within parentheses refer to 11-year-olds.

spective offered by the PG techniques, we hoped to bring into focus, step by step, some of the antecedent conditions in the genesis of anxiety, for without full knowledge of these conditions no therapeutic or preventive treatment can ever function to advantage.

SUBJECTS

NORMAL SCHOOLCHILDREN (AGE 7–15)

The main group of subjects consisted of 72 children from one school within the public school system in Lund.[2] A total of 37 girls and 35 boys were tested. Subjects were chosen so as to ensure an even distribution of the two sexes over age and a similarity in the proportion of children from "academic" (father holding a college degree) and nonacademic homes. About 40% of the children came from academic homes.

All subjects were presented with several Piagetian tasks. The

[2] Compulsory education begins at age 7 in Sweden.

landscape test served to differentiate between cognitively more and less mature children between 7 and 11 years (the task fails to differentiate above that age). The younger the children were, the more decisive the cognitive task was in placing them in the mature or immature age group (see Table 2.1). The 11-year-olds were divided into three groups, with the most mature ones (with no landscape errors) being included in the group of 12- to 13-year-olds.

YOUNG ADULTS (AGE 19)

Thirteen 19-year-old military conscripts served as an adult reference group for some of the MCT results. This group belonged to a larger one tested by Mrs. I. K. Nilsson for a different research purpose. About 30% of them came from academic homes; about 70% were still working to complete their education. We believe that intellectually this group does not deviate appreciably from the normal children.

A much larger adult reference group can be found in those subjects tested for previous studies using the MCT and AI test. This group primarily includes neurotic patients, with psychotic patients and normals also being represented.

CLINICAL CHILDREN (AGE 7-15)

The clinical group will be referred to only in passing. All subjects had been referred to us from a children's psychiatric clinic as patients presenting anxiety symptoms. Some of these children were considered to be near-psychotic.

The group included about 30 children. There were too few 7-and 8-year-olds to be of interest. In the age group 9–10(11), four of the 11 children belonged to the cognitively mature subgroup. Of the five (11)12- to 13-year-olds and ten 14- to 15-year-olds, four subjects (two in each group) were scored for errors on the landscape test. Thus, on the whole, the clinical children seemed to be cognitively somewhat more immature than their normal counterparts. As is often the case in a group of disturbed children, boys outnumbered girls (the ratio was about 2:1, whatever the age group).

All the clinical children were subjected to the same testing program as the normal ones, but some refused to take one or the other of the two PG tests.

METHOD

The MCT and the AI test have been described in Chapter 1. It should be pointed out that with the MCT we did not observe the subject's nonverbal behavior as closely and systematically as we did in the subsequent studies. Such observations are therefore not included in our data. For the landscape test, we placed the doll in only three of the viewing positions, excluding the child's own — a procedure different from that used with the preschool and the clinical children.

AFTERIMAGE TEST RESULTS

Already half a century ago it was demonstrated that positive and size-constant AIs are typical for children in contrast to adults (Kroh, 1922; Jaensch et al., 1929, 1930). Ruuth and Smith (1969) specifically demonstrated that these results correlated with signs of cognitive immaturity. They concluded "that resistance to an Emmert-type size increase is a sign of an incomplete objectivization (isolation) of the AI phenomenon; the positive hue can only be an additional sign of a preoperational confusion of AIs and real physical objects (stimulus)" (quoted in Andersson, Nilsson, Ruuth, and Smith, 1972, p. 108). To be sure, these primitive signs are not totally absent from the protocols of older children and are even scored in many adults, particularly in the early portions of their AI serials. Sudden appearances of size-constant or positive images in otherwise adult serials have been interpreted as regressions; they are typical of the AI protocols of acute schizophrenics (Smith, Ruuth, Franzén, and Sjöholm, 1972).

Our AI results are summarized in Tables 2.2–2.4, where S represents AI size, and I represents the intensity estimate. The scoring principles were adopted from previous studies. An AI

≤ 6.5 cm was thus considered size-constant. Positive images could be red, orange, violet, yellow, and/or very bright ($I = 1$–2, when relatively dark hues were expected following a bright stimulus). Among the positive images, we distinguished between entirely positive, stable ones and only partly positive (variegated) AIs or AIs fluctuating between positive and negative colors. The particular meaning of variegated and fluctuating AIs will be discussed later.

Table 2.2 shows very clearly that the relative number of subjects with primitive AI signs diminishes with increased age and cognitive maturity. Size-constant AIs tend to disappear faster than positive ones. A size-constant image appears to be a more obvious sign of immature cognitive functioning, of an inability clearly to distinguish between what comes from the self and what occurs in an independent outside world. It should be added that subjects with entirely size-constant and/or positive AIs are rarely found outside the youngest and most immature children.

Distinctly green AIs have been listed as a separate category in Table 2.2. They have repeatedly proved to be signs of compulsive tendencies. In one AI experiment a subliminal threat was administered to arouse anxiety (Andersson, Fries, and Smith, 1970). When a green color was reported (instead of the expected bluish or even black anxiety hue), this was interpreted as follows: "The reported clarity of the color . . . tends to enhance isolation of the 'subjective' image from the 'real' perceptual environment and to mark its nonthreatening character. Thus the green image, even if more intense than previous images, usually does not appear darker and does not enlarge beyond its initially established boundaries" (Andersson, Nilsson, Ruuth, and Smith, 1972, p. 100). In other words, the green color serves as a protection against the tendency of the AI to darken (become oversaturated) and to grow during states of anxiety (see below). We shall discuss later the definite accumulation of green or green-spotted images during prepuberty, in the group (11)12–13 years.

The last column in Table 2.2 summarizes the number of variegated AIs and AIs fluctuating between different colors (shifts between red, green, and blue hues occurring the most

TABLE 2.2
PRIMITIVE AI SIGNS AND GREEN COLOR

Group	I≥2 positive (uniform, stable)	I≥1 positive (variegated, fluctuating)	I≥2 S≤6.5	I≥2 uniform, positive or small	I≥1 green (uniform, stable)	I≥1 green (variegated, fluctuating)	I≥1 green (all)	I≥1 variegated or with chromatic fluctuation
7–8 immature	2	0	3	5	1	0	1	0
7–8 mature	4 — 15 (19)	1	2 — 10 (24)	5 — 10 (4)*	3	2	4 — 10 (24)	2 — 5 (29)
9–10(11) immature	4	2	4	6 — 11 (9)	3	1	4	2
9–10(11) mature	5	1	1	5	1	0	1	1
(11)12–13	6 — 12 (24)	7	1 — 2 (34)	6 — 13 (23)	7	4	10 — 15 (21)	8 — 14 (22)
14–15	6	6	1	7	3	2	5	6

* Figures within parentheses represent the remaining number of subjects.

often). A special investigation has established significant correlations between these signs and hypersensitivity or projective tendencies (Smith, Sjöholm, and Nielzén, 1974). The authors conclude that "the particular kind of AI coloring . . . reflects a specific relation between the individual and his perceived world, a relation leading to subjective involvement and uncertainty (or particular concern about these matters)" (p. 46). In our study there seems to be an increase in the number of variegated or fluctuating AIs in the older age groups, indicating a less immediate dependence on the stimulus.

Size-constant and very large AIs (≥ 11.0 cm) often appear in the same protocol, suggesting a general uncertainty about the relation between subjective and objective variables in the perceptual field. Here we might expect size-constant AIs mixed with enlarged ones to be more common than size-constant AIs alone in children who are no longer totally enclosed in their egocentric thinking but have begun to glimpse a world of independent relationships (Ruuth, 1970; Ruuth and Andersson, 1971). These children's first attempts to adapt to the geometric principles reflected in Emmert's law would, naturally, be exaggerated. These speculations are to some extent supported by the data in Table 2.3. Although size deviations are generally more common in the younger age groups, size constancy seems to be the most typical deviation of the very young children. As will be discussed, protocols with enlarged AIs but no size-constant AIs present their own problems.

Anxiety is indicated in adult AI protocols by enlarged and dark (most often achromatic) images (Andersson, Nilsson, Ruuth, and Smith, 1972). In a factor analysis of results from a moderately depressed patient group, positive AIs also clustered in the anxiety factor (Smith, Fries, Andersson, and Ried, 1971). Red color (like other primitive signs) supposedly signified a mobilization of defensive measures (regression). More recent studies have found that the total absence of AIs in a serial also denotes anxiety (e.g., Smith and Sjöholm, 1974b; Smith, Sjöholm, and Nielzén, 1975, 1976).

The anxiety signs shown to be useful in adults, however, could not necessarily be trusted in children. We did not score large AIs as anxiety signs in protocols revealing an uncertain

Table 2.3
AI Size Estimates

Group	At least two deviations				Single deviations			Rest of sample
	$S \leq 6.5$	$S \leq 6.5$ and $S \geq 11.0$	$S \geq 11.0$	Σ	$S \leq 6.5$	$S \geq 11.0$	Σ	
7–8 immature	2	1	2	5	0	0	0	2
7–8 mature	1	2	1	4	0	0	0	2
9–10(11) immature	2	2	1	5	0	3	3	2
9–10(11) mature	0	1	1	2	1	2	3	5
(11)12–13	1	0	2	3	1	1	2	11
14–15	1	2	1	4	2	1	3	12

Paired totals (brackets): 7–8 group Σ = 9, Single = 0, Rest = 4; 9–10(11) group Σ = 7, Single = 6, Rest = 7; (11)12–15 group Σ = 7, Single = 5, Rest = 23.

grasp of the relation between the AI and perceived reality, i.e., in subjects with size-constant images. Nor did we find the presence of primitive AIs useful for the youngest and most immature groups (although it did differentiate in the two oldest ones). Because of these expected deficiencies in reliability, the scoring rules for anxiety signs in children were strengthened (see Table 2.4). One exception was that the usual size limit for large AIs (11.0 cm) was lowered to 10.5 cm in order to include a number of children with such slightly smaller AIs. Since, for the reasons just discussed, the same scoring principles could not be used for all subjects, comparisons between age and cognitive maturity levels should be made with caution. Nevertheless, our impression is that in the oldest (puberty) group more subjects showed anxiety than in the other groups (see also the right column in Table 2.4, where subjects with adult anxiety signs are listed).

It may also be instructive to cite a few findings from the two largest subgroups of the clinical subjects. Six of the 11 clinical subjects in the age group 9–10(11) years were scored for large AIs and/or for a loss of more than two phases, compared with only five of the 20 normals in the corresponding age group. Similarly, in the age group 14–15 years, six of the 10 clinical subjects were scored for these signs, whereas five of the 19 normal children were so scored. We should also note that the remaining four clinical subjects were all scored for primitive AIs. Three of them had primitive AIs in as many as nine or 10 phases, while none of the six normal subjects with primitive AIs showed such a high frequency. These differences are enhanced if scoring is restricted to manifest anxiety signs, i.e., to signs appearing in the last half of the AI serial. However, since we shortened the number of trials with our children, we cannot be sure, particularly with the older children, who may adapt more slowly, that late scores always represent a C-phase level. We shall therefore not stress this particular point.

We shall now follow this perusal of the main tendencies evident in our AI data with a more specific discussion of the relationships between the AI and MCT results. Both tests will help us to characterize the developmental trends in the present group of children.

TABLE 2.4
ANXIETY SIGNS IN AI TEST

Group	S At least 3S≥10.5 (not in unstable serials)	I At least 2I (achr.) ≥10*	S + I At least 1I (achr.) ≥10	Single 2S/11 (achr.) ≥10*	Loss of >2 phases	Primitive (≥5 phases with primitive signs)	Adult signs (some S≥11.0 or I [achr.] ≥10)	N
7–8 immature	2	2	0	2	2	–	–	9
7–8 mature	1	1	0	3	0	–	–	7
9–10(11) immature	0	0	2	2	0	–	–	10
9–10(11) mature	0	2	1	2	0	–	–	10
(11)12–13	1	2	1	5	1	4**	6	17
14–15	1	4	0	3	0	6**	10	19

* Or 2 I (achr.) = 9, or 3 I (chr.) ≥10, instead of 1 I (achr.) ≥10.
** If the subjects already scored in the left columns are discounted, the figures change to 3 and 4, respectively.

Meta-Contrast Technique Results

Anxiety

In a series of investigations with adults (see Smith, Sjöholm, and Nielzén, 1975, 1976), the following major types of anxiety signs have been established: (1) *weakening of defense structures* (e.g., the disappearance of a white screen erected to isolate the hero in B_2 from the threatening A_2); (2) *disintegration of the stabilized perceptual frame* (e.g., the B picture [even B_1] becomes less clear or is even partially lost); and (3) *dark structures* (e.g., a black wall behind the hero or a threatening night sky outside the window).

We used the AI results to test these signs in the present sample. As mentioned in Chapter 1, AI data have proved to be quite effective in spotting anxiety in adult subjects. The necessary adjustments in the AI scoring dimensions for children have just been discussed. After making these corrections, we found enough difference between normal and clinical children to warrant using the AI data as anxiety criteria, at least tentatively.

The adult anxiety signs in the MCT (described above) did not, however, correlate very well with the AI signs, particularly not in the youngest children. Several factors may account for this. It seems reasonable to assume that defense structures are not as firmly established in children as in adults. The child's perceptual world is generally less stable; it is more likely to change from one form of organization to another. Therefore, intermittent structural disintegrations scored in the MCT would be less significant in children than in adults. Moreover, we also have to consider that a child's anxiety tends to be expressed in a way directly related to the concrete situation (phobic fear instead of signal anxiety). As we have stated, according to psychoanalytic theory, the infant's primary anxiety reactions are directly tied to the stimulus context and appear more or less automatically on the loss of a need-satisfying object. The use of anxiety as a danger signal presupposes the ability to anticipate a dreaded situation and must therefore be a more advanced reaction (Freud, 1926; Edgcumbe and Burgner, 1972).

With these considerations in mind, we looked, first of all, for *pronounced breakdowns* of established structures, such as the total disappearance of a meaningful B (*zero-phases*) or the disappearance of the hero in B_2 (here we are not referring to a neglect to report the hero but to an active assertion that he is absent). We also noticed an inability clearly to extricate the self from a dangerous situation, which was expressed in a *fusion of the hero and the threat.* Sometimes the child saw them very close together; at other times he was unable to distinguish between them.[3] It should be noted that this kind of fusion is not a necessary consequence of cognitive immaturity. Rather, in emphasizing signs of fusion, we have in mind such early disturbances in the sense of reality and identity as have been linked by Greenacre (1967) and others to a predisposition to anxiety. We thus assumed that a child who could not keep the threat at arm's length from the hero would probably lack the ability to cope with danger signals and to preserve an inner sense of security. As might be expected, these two kinds of MCT anxiety signs are typical of the younger children, in whom they are clearly associated with AI anxiety signs (see Table 2.5 and our later discussion of its significance).

In the two upper age groups, *dark structures,* particularly if they appear in the last third of the A + B section (close to the C-phase), are the most prominent anxiety signs. Moreover, in these older youngsters, *structural disintegration,* another sign in adults, also seems to have some validity. *Phobic features* in advanced forms (reports of objects in the window which are very different from A_2) are also worth paying attention to because in other studies they have been associated with anxiety hysteria, in particular. *Direct expressions of fright* have often been noted in adult groups but could not be scored with certainty here.

A few additional data may be of interest. With the AI results, we noted that anxiety signs seem more common in early adolescence (14–15 years) than in prepuberty ([11]12–13 years). This

---

[3] A few tentative reports of fusion were followed, not later than the next phase, by assertions that A_2 and the hero had nothing to do with each other, or the like. These reports were not scored.

TABLE 2.5
ANXIETY SIGNS IN AI TEST AND MCT

MCT Signs	AI Signs			
	S/I/Loss	Primitive	Single	Rest of sample
Age 7–10(11)				
Strong				
Zero-phase/hero disappearance	4	–	0	1
Fusion	6	– Σ10	1 Σ1	1 Σ2
Medium				
Dark structures	2	–	2	3
Broken structures	1	–	0	0
Advanced phobic features	0	– Σ3	1 Σ3	0 Σ3
Weak				
Structural disintegration	0	–	1	0
Diffusion	0	–	0	3
No signs	1	– Σ1	5 Σ6	4 Σ7
Age 11(12–15)				
Strong				
Fusion	1	0	0	1
Late dark structures	3	4	0	1
Advanced phobic features	3	2 Σ13	0 Σ0	0 Σ2
Medium				
Early dark structures	1	1	1	2
Structural disintegration	2	0	0	2
Broken structures	0	0 Σ4	2 Σ3	0 Σ4
Weak				
No signs	0	2 Σ2	2 Σ2	6 Σ6

impression is corroborated by the MCT results. Whereas 12 (of 19) 14- to 15-year-olds were scored for dark structures, only five (of 17) subjects in the prepuberty group were. In the older group, reports of fusion occurred twice (against zero times in the younger one) and reports of diffusion six times (against only once in the younger group). In the group of 13 conscripts the number of subjects scored for darkness was lower (three), as one would expect. The other anxiety signs in this group, although typically adult, also occurred less frequently, with only two scores for structural disintegration and one for diffusion.

As with the AI results, we shall make a tentative comparison with the clinical group, excluding the 7- to 8-year-olds. Only manifest signs have been marked, i.e., signs appearing in the last third of the A + B section. Ten of the 24 clinical subjects but none of the 56 normals aged 9 to 15 showed late zero-phases, fusion, or expressions of fright. Late dark structures were scored in three additional clinical subjects (making nine cases altogether) and in 14 normal subjects. The anxiety signs most typical of the clinical children — zero-phases and fusion — were not only absent from the late phases of percept genesis in all normal subjects but were almost totally absent in the two oldest age groups (cf. the thoroughly primitivized AI serials in some clinical youngsters).

Primitive Mechanisms

The most convenient way for a child at the egocentric cognitive level to avoid threatening realities is to deny them by simply not looking. In line with this, *eye shutting by the hero* (or head turning, etc.) is the most common defensive tactic in the youngest and most cognitively immature age group (see Table 2.6). These subjects do not shut their own eyes (as immature preschool subjects may do) but report that the hero closes his eyes or turns his gaze away from the window. This kind of representational avoidance strategy, which implies elimination of all conceivably dangerous information, seems akin to descriptions of denial by child analysts.

We shall see below that older children report, not the hero's turning away from A_2, but A_2's turning his back on the hero. The youngest and most immature children are not very likely to be scored for this kind of defense. As a matter of fact, eye shutting by the hero and turning the threat's head away are only rarely scored in the same protocol and do not appear together in young children. A prerequisite for the use of the latter strategy would be a less egocentric cognitive outlook, implying that the world does not cease to exist because you refuse to look at it (see the discussion of compulsive mechanisms below).

In the MCT manual (Smith, Johnsson, Ljunghill-Andersson, and Almgren, 1970), a number of signs appear under the heading *repression*. They include reports not only of

TABLE 2.6
EYE SHUTTING (ES) BY THE HERO AND HERO DUPLICATION (HD) IN MCT

Group	Many phases directly before C (or uninterrupted continuity)		Many phases followed by turning away, etc., within the theme	Many phases followed by other defenses		Single phase		Σ with such defenses	Σ without them
	ES	HD	HD	ES	HD	ES	HD		
7–8 immature	3*	5	0	1	0	1	0	9	0
7–8 mature	0	1	0	0	0	0	1	2	5
9–10(11) immature	0	2	2	0	1	3	0	6	4
9–10(11) mature	0	0	1	0	0	1	1	3	7
(11)12–13	0	0	0	0	2	0	2	4	13
14–15	0	0	1	1	0	1	1	4	15

* In one subject eye shutting by the hero and hero duplication coincide in one phase.

busts or masks instead of A_2, but also of torn-off body parts, nondangerous animals, trees, and even stimulus-distant objects (a house, a radio, a bicycle). These transformations of the threat into something stiff, limp, or hollow, into a plaything or a lifeless object, have proved to be typical of hysterics, with the more stimulus-distant interpretations found most often in anxiety hysterics and phobics. The association between primitive hysteria or anxiety hysteria and this class of signs was the main reason for calling them repressive.

TABLE 2.7
SIGNS OF REPRESSION IN MCT

Group	a No signs	b Protocols with torn-off body parts	c Others, lacking b but with masks or objects	d Others, lacking b and c but with animals, trees, etc.
7–8 immature	4	4	0	1
7–8 mature	4	0	3	0
9–10(11) immature	4	2	4	0
9–10(11) mature	3	3	2	2
(11)12–13	5	2	6	4
14–15	8	1	7	3

Looking at the signs of repression listed in Table 2.7, one detects a change over age in the balance between them. Reports of torn-off body parts are relatively common in young and cognitively immature children; in older children they are replaced by reports of lifeless masks or objects. (Note that none of the immature 7- to 8-year-olds reported lifeless masks or objects.) Taking all the so-called phobic (stimulus-distant) signs (objects, trees, etc.), we find they occur in 18 of 36 protocols in the two older groups but in only three of 16 protocols in the 7- to 8-year-olds.

Repression is supposed to be an early form of defense. Insofar as our different signs reflect the same basic tactic of repression, it appears to be a strategy that can be adapted to the increasing sophistication of the growing child. To change a threatening face into a tree, and, even more, to change it into a lifeless object, is clearly a more advanced and active form of disarming a threat than merely to ignore everything except an ear, a piece of hair, or another isolated area of the head. The last, primitive kind of repression bears an obvious resemblance to eye shutting by the hero,—and to denial.

Another form of defense in young children is termed *hero duplication*. By this we mean casting A_2 in the form of the hero in B_2 or, more concretely, placing a reflection of the hero or a playmate approximately his age in the window. To couch this in the language of the representational world (Sandler and Rosenblatt, 1962), in hero duplication the subject appears to invest his self-representation with the power of the representatives of the outside, threatening world. Such a response is, in any case, a primitive, narcissistic form of avoidance.

It is particularly revealing, and consonant with the assumptions of PG theory, that both eye shutting by the hero and hero duplication appear very close to the C-phase in the youngest and most immature groups (see Table 2.6 and Figure 2.1). Eventually, these responses are pushed back from the C-phase, and other forms of defense come to the fore. From a PG perspective, one can say that, as children grow, manifest (primitive) mechanisms become more and more latent and finally disappear as other contents crowd the PG process. The eye-shutting response disappears more rapidly with increasing age and is presumably more primitive than hero duplication. It is, however, more sophisticated than eye-shutting *behavior* (shutting one's own eyes), which we noted in children younger than those tested here (see Chapter 3). Among the 13 conscripts, there was only one, uncertain case of hero duplication. But 14 of the 24 clinical subjects (excluding the youngest ones) used this primitive device, compared with 13 of the 56 normal children in the corresponding age groups. It is still used by close to half of the clinical 14- to 15-year-olds.

In some adults one finds repeated, stereotypic reports of a split B_2 stimulus (e.g., the window is seen before the rest of the picture), instead of A_2 preceding B_2. Such signs of *primitive stereotypy* were typical for a group of "accident-loaded," as opposed to "accident-free," car drivers (Andersson, Nilsson, and Hen-

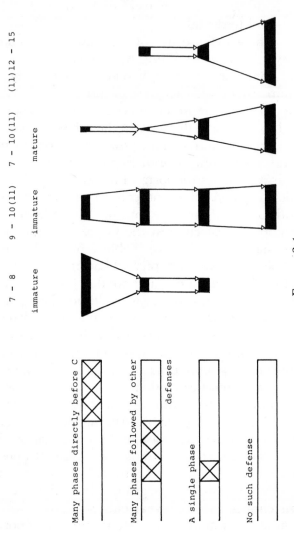

FIGURE 2.1

PROPORTION OF EYE SHUTTING BY THE HERO AND HERO DUPLICATION IN MCT.

riksson, 1970). According to these investigators, "the splitting seems to indicate that the subject avoids being conscious of 'anxiety', provoked by the . . . 'threat' . . . by utilizing extraceptive perception of a part of the B-stimulus (the window)" (p. 416). This stereotypic dependence on extraceptive factors was not found in a single child but showed up in a few of the 19-year-old conscripts. In some way, however, hero duplication also reflects a dependence on outside factors in the child's attempts to avert the threat. Even if it is true that most reports of hero duplication are not stereotyped (a lively interaction between the hero and his duplicate is often described), traces of beginning stereotypy or formalism can be observed in some protocols.

In discussing the anxiety signs, we assumed that the perceptual world of the child would be less stable than that of the adult. Young children are more likely than older ones suddenly to lose either the hero or a correctly recognized A_2. We found four such cases among the 16 children aged 7 to 8, compared with only three among the remaining 56 children. More subtle signs of an unstable C-phase were distributed in a similar way.

Another interesting characteristic in young children's reports is termed *retention*. It is scored when a child offers a new interpretation in phase N, but at the same time holds onto the interpretation given in phase $N-1$, thus balancing two or more meanings against each other. Stimulus A_2 may, for instance, first be reported as a blackbird. The next report may describe A_2 as a person, but the blackbird does not disappear—both are seen together. Children showing retention do not eliminate P-phase contents—as an adult would—but carry along early, stimulus-distant meanings in the process of percept construction. In 36 protocols from the four youngest groups, 14 cases of retention were found; in the 36 remaining protocols, only two.

The use of *alternative interpretations* seems to be more common than retention in older children. Seven such cases were scored in the two oldest groups and six in the younger children. This sign does not imply the simultaneous reporting of many competing meanings (as when the blackbird and person appeared together), but rather the possibility of choice: "It could either be a blackbird or a human being." Alternative interpretations would represent a more mature way of reconstructing the ambiguity and condensation of early phases in percept genesis.

It is natural to think of retention and alternative interpretations as reflecting a high degree of freedom of communication between various phases, early and late, in the PG process. Such freedom may be one important prerequisite for creativity. A characteristic of our clinical children was the lack of this freedom. Only two of the 24 older clinical subjects were scored for retention or alternative interpretations, compared with 16 of the 56 older normal subjects.

COMPULSIVE MECHANISMS

An imposing display of reactions have been assembled under the general heading *compulsive mechanisms*. Among the valid signs of compulsive symptoms in adults, we particularly wish to mention *negation* ("it is not a threatening face") and *isolation* (reports that A_2 is a clean white surface, that is separated from the hero by a barrier, or that curtains cover the window). In *empty serials* no changes are reported until A_2 emerges as the correct percept. Here we should also note *perceptual manipulations* (descriptions of small changes, most often in or around the window) and *intellectualization* (the threat is classed as a mere fantasy or thought product). The most important strategy in this category, however, is *turning away the head of the threat*. Not only have reports of the back of a head been scored but also reports of a profile turned away from the hero.

Excluding from consideration here the two younger age groups (in which compulsive signs are rare), if we take green color for granted as a compulsive sign in the AI test, then turning away seems to be its most obvious counterpart in the MCT (see Table 2.8 and our later discussion of its significance). Other signs of compulsive strategies appear to be less clear-cut, unless they are combined with turning away. The compulsive mechanisms in adults listed above may appear as more general signs of avoidance behavior in children. Only in grownups, however, do these tactics signify a typically compulsive defense. Moreover, we may not even be able to take the meaning of green AI color for granted in children. Nor do we know for sure that the absence of large-sized or very dark AIs are medium-

TABLE 2.8

COMPULSIVE SIGNS IN AI TEST AND MCT (9- TO 15-YEAR-OLDS)

AI Signs	MCT Signs						
	Turning away without isolation/ negation	Turning away with isolation/ negation	Σ	Isolation/ negation/ empty serials	Isolation (only empty faces)	Σ	Rest of sample
Some clearly green AIs	9	5	14 (10)*	4	1	5 (5)	0 (0)
All S< 10/all I< 9	4	6	10 (6)	3	3	6 (5)	3 (3)
The rest	5	1	6 (1)	5	2	7 (4)	4 (2)

* Figures within parentheses refer to the two oldest age groups.

strong compulsive signs in children, although that seems to be the case in adults (see Table 2.8).

Turning away often grows out of the primitive mechanism of hero duplication, i.e., the duplicate hero in the window starts turning his head away from the observer (Table 2.9). This change may signify a waning of the duplication strategy. In older children turning away becomes a mechanism in its own right but is more and more supplemented by isolation in its mature forms (separating the threat and the hero, whitewashing, etc.). It should be noted that turning away was found in four of the 13 conscripts.

The peak age for all the "compulsive" defenses (turning away, negation, isolation, intellectualization, perceptual manipulation) was (11)12–13 years. If we exclude reports of empty faces (one of the least specific signs of compulsion, to judge from Table 2.8), eight of these 17 youngsters were scored for isolation, compared with four of the children aged 14–15. At the same time anxiety signs proved to be relatively sparse. According to our data, then, prepuberty is not an age of low emotional tide but a period when emotions are actively warded off in order to promote adaptation to external realities. One might also speak of a consolidation in preparation for the emotional convulsions of puberty and adolescence. We intend to return to this age group later. Let us only note here that such a conclusion is entirely in line with the writings of Anna Freud (1936, 1965).

A special defense comes to the fore at the height of puberty: reports of an A_2 lacking recognizable features. It may be difficult for younger children to use this rather sophisticated defensive measure because lack of features would in itself be anxiety-provoking for them. However, this particular defense appears to peak at age 14–15, with nine scored cases out of 19. In the conscript group we find only two protocols marked for it.

As we have seen, turning away and other "compulsive" defenses appear to be more frequent in the older age groups than in the young ones. Since the clinical subjects were characterized by primitive expressions of anxiety as well as by the use of such primitive defenses as hero duplication, we did not expect a high frequency for turning away in this group. Only seven (of 24) clinical children employed this threat-

TABLE 2.9

TURNING AWAY OF THREAT IN MCT

Group	Manifested only within hero duplication	More unclear combination with hero duplication*	Combined with repression	No such combination		Σ Presence	Σ Absence
				Directly before C-phase	Followed by negation, isolation, intellectualization, etc.		
7–8 immature	1	0	0	0	0	1	8
7–8 mature	1	1	0	0	0	2	5
9–10(11) immature	3	1	2	0	0	6	4
9–10(11) mature	2	0	2	2	1	7	3
(11)12–13	0	1	1	6	1	9	8
14–15	0	0	0	4	4	8	11

* Begins in hero duplication; concerns hero's mother; shifting between hero and threat.

averting method, compared with 30 (of 56) normal subjects. Simple devices like turning away may be an important piece of defensive equipment for the normal post-egocentric child, just as eye shutting by the hero or total denial is a necessary defense for the normal egocentric child.

HYPERSENSITIVITY AND PROJECTION

In cases of hypersensitivity, instead of establishing itself as an independent perception, A makes itself felt through changes in the B-percept. In other words, contents outside the subject's immediate awareness are "projected" onto his established perceptual world. Common signs of oversensitivity are shifts in the lighting or position of the furniture (in B_1) and the hero (in B_2), changes not reported in the control series (where B was not yet preceded by A). The B-changes scored as hypersensitive are not so profound as to endanger the subject's belief that B is essentially the same stimulus from one exposure to the next. Major projective changes are scored as discontinuities.

Hypersensitivity has proved to be a positive diagnostic sign in adults (Smith, Sjöholm, and Nielzén, 1975), implying a readiness to register even marginal internal or external cues and to change accordingly. More marked signs of projection, such as drastic change in B or the introduction of new persons, carry a rather negative prognosis and often correlate with paranoid inflexibility. What we have scored as projective tendencies in children are nowhere near these extreme projections in adults. Reports of movement and of interaction between the hero and the threat do not, however, belong to exactly the same category as hypersensitivity and should be treated separately. They seem to reflect a greater degree of self-indulgence in the treatment of outside information.

The scoring of hypersensitivity and mild projection may be affected by the momentary whims of a subject. In order to enhance the reliability in adult subjects, we have required that these tendencies be scored in at least two phases. Expecting even lower reliability in children than in adults, we also excluded subjects with obvious tendencies to manipulate perceptual details, i.e., subjects who in their manipulation of outside stimulation tend to handle it in an inflexible, controlling manner.

In view of previous research (Smith, Sjöholm, and Nielzén, 1974), hypersensitivity should correlate above all with AI variegation and within-phase chromatic shifts. In Table 2.10 we have included not only a chromatic shift within or between phases but also its counterpart in the size dimension (when serials are chromatically stable): change between size-constant and at least normal-size AIs. Correlations in the expected direction are evident.

There is a weak trend toward increased sensitivity in puberty compared with the younger age groups. Five of the 19 pubescent adolescents were scored for hypersensitivity but only seven of the 53 others. If alternative interpretations and hypersensitivity are both interpreted as signs of readiness to accept change, 10 out of 19 pubescent subjects show such readiness but only four of 17 prepubescent ones.

The mood of the hero in B_2 as reported by the child was also scored, but no age tendencies could be detected. Reports of a depressed hero are discussed in the next section.

Deviant Reactions

Under this heading we have listed various reactions which are relatively rare among normal children but are often encountered in the clinical group. Some of these reactions are well known from our investigations of adult patients.

Breaks in the continuity of percept construction occurred in 11 of the 24 clinical subjects over age 8. This scoring category encompasses zero-phases (at least two), loss of the hero in the established B-percept, loss of a correct A, and structural change implying a return to previously discarded interpretations (regression). In the corresponding age group of 56 normals, only three subjects showed these signs. It has already been noted that the C-phase is less stable in children under 9 years of age. Using the above guidelines, we can score five of our 16 normal 7- to 8-year-olds for breaks in continuity.

Another category includes *depressive or empty protocols*. A depressive serial is often stereotyped, with at least five unchanged repetitions of an "unfinished" interpretation of A. Another

TABLE 2.10
HYPERSENSITIVITY AND PROJECTION IN AI TEST AND MCT

MCT Signs	AI Signs		
	Variegation/chromatic within-phase change	Chromatic between-phase change/size instability (at least 2 phases)	Rest of sample
Hypersensitivity (not perceptual manipulation)	6	4	2
Movement, interaction, projection (not perceptual manipulation)	4	2	5
Hypersensitivity, movement, etc. + perceptual manipulation	3	2	5
Rest of sample	6	7	24

sign of depression is the description of A_2 as very old, weak, sick, or dead. We have also included protocols where the hero is described as clearly grief-stricken and depressed. In empty protocols, as already noted, only B is reported and nothing appears to change or develop until a correct A suddenly emerges. Empty protocols have been recorded not only in compulsive but also in depressed patients. We counted 16 depressed or empty protocols in each of the groups compared (the 24 clinical and 56 normal subjects).

One of our most interesting discoveries is the existence of *leaking mechanisms* in 13 of the 24 clinical subjects over age 8. This designation applies when, in the same phase, a subject shows both a defensive strategy (most often compulsive or repressive) and signs of anxiety (mainly dark structures). A child may transform the threatening A_2 into a lifeless mask, but a mask reflecting blackness. Apparently, his defense is not efficient, for the "black" of anxiety "leaks" through. Only seven normals in the group of 56 were (rather liberally) scored for these mechanisms. One of the reasons why normal children appear to be more tolerant of a certain amount of anxiety than many clinical children may be a basic trust in their own ability to curb it effectively when necessary.

The difference between a deviant MCT protocol and a more normal one is schematically illustrated in Figures 2.2 and 2.3.

AGE AND COGNITIVE MATURITY GROUPS

The following description of the age and cognitive maturity groups in the normal sample is based on the main AI and MCT results. It has already been shown that these two instruments correlate along measures of analogous personality dimensions.

AGE 7–8 YEARS: IMMATURE

This group was the most P-phase-dominated. In five of seven children with measurable AIs, at least two phases were characterized by size constancy or by positive color (covering

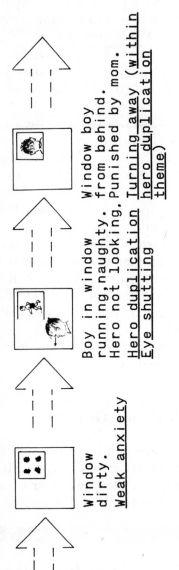

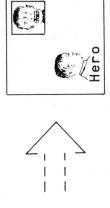

FIGURE 2.2

SCHEMATICALLY ILLUSTRATED EXCERPTS FROM THE MCT PROTOCOL
OF A 9-YEAR-OLD, COGNITIVELY MATURE, NORMAL GIRL.

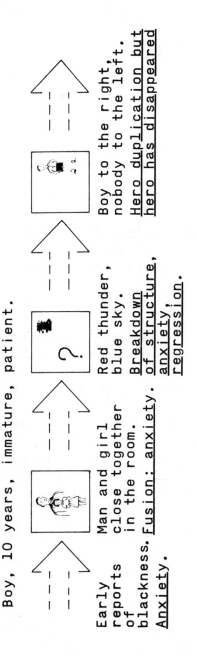

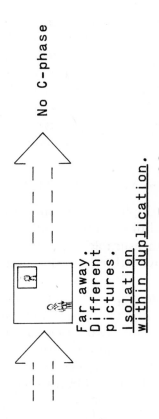

FIGURE 2.3

SCHEMATICALLY ILLUSTRATED EXCERPTS FROM THE MCT PROTOCOL
OF A 10-YEAR-OLD, COGNITIVELY IMMATURE BOY IN THE CLINICAL GROUP.

the entire image). Many serials did not contain any negative (chromatic) images. Five of nine MCT protocols were scored for retention (i.e., these children did not eliminate early P-phase formations but tended to carry them along in the process of percept construction).

The defense mechanisms elucidated by the MCT were on the whole primitive and narcissistic. Eye shutting by the hero was reported by three children right up to the C-phase and hero duplication by five children. All members of this group were scored for one or both of these mechanisms. Turning-away responses and isolation, on the other hand, occurred only in single protocols and intellectualization not at all. Repression appeared in its most primitive form—with reports of fragmented body parts, similar to partial denial.

Another primitive characteristic was that these children's adaptive processes often lacked stable end-stages: three children were scored for an unstable C-phase and four for discontinuity.

Age 7–8 Years: Mature

The P-phase dominance was only beginning to abate in this young but cognitively advanced group. Five of seven children with measurable AIs still received at least two scores for primitive AI signs. But green color was reported by three children. Three of seven children were characterized by unstable C-phases and four by discontinuity. However, eye shutting by the hero did not appear, and hero duplication was seen in only two cases (and in one of these, just in a single phase). Compulsive trends, however, had begun to assert themselves, as shown by four cases of isolation and two of intellectualization. On the other hand, it should be noted that the turning-away defense (two cases) was still closely tied to its primitive precursors (hero duplication).

Age 9–10(11) Years: Immature

This group was quite similar to the immature 7- to 8-year-olds. There were still plenty of primitive AIs (in six of 10 children) and primitive defensive measures (five children with hero duplication and three with single scores for eye shutting by the hero). But it was no longer sufficient for the subject to place a duplicate of the hero in the window; the head of the duplicate had to be turned away in order for the defense to be effective. Apparently, this more sophisticated mode of avoidance still originated in more primitive methods (four started with hero duplication and two with repression). The group also differed from both of the younger groups in its greater perceptual stability (only two children were scored for unstable C-phases and one for discontinuity).

Age 9–10(11) Years: Mature

C-phase dominance steadily increased. It is true that half of the 10 children showed primitive AI signs. The AIs, however, were mostly of normal size, and positive series were interspersed not with achromatic AIs but with negatives ones. Turning away became a more frequent defense (seven children) and was less often tied to hero duplication (two children). While three subjects were scored for hero duplication (and only one for more than one phase), five were scored for isolation. The elimination of P-phase formations in the MCT was still incomplete, with five cases of retention.

Age (11)12–13 Years

Among all the groups in the study, this one was clearly the most C-phase-dominated. The primitive AI signs noted in the younger age groups could be found in six of 17 subjects, but size constancy in only one. Instead of positive color entirely covering the AI, a change to color-spotted AIs seemed to take place (eight subjects). Retention did not occur in a single child, nor did late hero duplication.

The greater reality orientation of this group seemed to be effected in part by compulsive defenses. Ten children were scored for green AI color, nine for turning away, and ten for isolation. More sophisticated and active forms of repression also asserted themselves. The anxiety level was judged as relatively low, at least in the MCT.

According to the test data, this appears to be an age of extroversion and consolidation. Functionally speaking, this may be seen as a preparatory stage for the renewed reconstruction of P-phase formations in puberty; it is a stage where the C-phase is above all strengthened. At the same time, there is a growing independence from the immediate stimulus situation, as evidenced by a sudden increase in variegated AIs.

AGE 14–15 YEARS

Although C-phase stability was maintained, a new reconstruction of P-phase formations was apparent. Positive AIs occurred in six of 19 cases (but only one showed size constancy); variegated or fluctuating AIs with red color appeared in six cases. But the number of "green" protocols dropped to five. Even in the MCT, there was a slight drop in the number of turning-away scores (eight) and still more in the number of "true" isolation scores (four against eight in the preceding group, not counting faces without features).

At the same time, the number of scores for dark structures changed in the opposite direction (from five to 12). AI data show an increase in the proportion of adult anxiety signs, with hypersensitivity signs at a high level. In the MCT hypersensitivity and alternative interpretations seem to be more frequent in this group (10 children, compared with four youngsters in the preceding group). This finding was interpreted as indicating the adolescent's greater willingness to accept change and to harbor contradictory meanings.

Relaxing their defensive barriers, these young adolescents are apparently ready to face new adaptive demands. They even seem ready to tolerate more anxiety as a consequence. An important prerequisite for this openness and independence appears to be a stable C-phase level, acquired during prepuberty.

DISCUSSION

In PG research, where children report their impressions of very brief exposures or where the attempt is made to measure and describe elusive AI phenomena, the issue of reliability must be considered. Presuming that children's reports are inevitably less reliable than those of adults, we applied stricter scoring rules and were especially on guard against any tendency to give vague and ambivalent utterances a "fitting" interpretation. Here it should be noted that results from other studies agree well with our findings (Lindbom, 1968; Andersson, Nilsson, Ruuth, and Smith, 1972), or with what could generally be expected of these age groups. It should also be pointed out that unreliable data would not usually yield a systematic pattern of "false" differences but a mess of unsystematic and weak differences.

If we wished to improve the reliability of our data, why did we choose to work with a relatively limited number of subjects? More material would undoubtedly have afforded a better opportunity to observe less prominent trends, despite the background noise insufficient reliability represents. We have, however, always been wary of those diffuse tendencies obtained with extensive data collection — so overexploited in behavioral research — which only just manage to ripple the probability surface. Instead, we found a medium sample size more conducive to careful scrutiny of each individual protocol. Large data accumulations are seldom amenable to anything but the most conventional handling. In the present study this would have meant scoring children's protocols according to the rules already established for adults.

The group of normal children studied here is obviously not socially or intellectually representative. Our intention was not to set up age norms but only to follow development over age. The requirements of such a study have been met by careful matching of sex and intellectual background in the four age groups. Naturally, when age groups were broken up into cognitive maturity levels, the balance between academic and nonacademic families sometimes collapsed.

The group of clinical children used here is deficient in many ways. First of all, there are too few young children. Yet the lopsided age distribution in a sense reflects the general fears and aversions of clinical children, evident above all in the youngest children's refusal to participate in any testing program, at least when they do not know the experimenter well. Second, the single characteristic used to select the group was anxiety — any symptoms of anxiety. Because of these limitations, the clinical group served only as a contrasting backdrop for the normal group. It allowed us to generate hypotheses requiring further, more specific studies of anxiety and defense against anxiety in children.

No p-values are given in the comparisons in the tables of this first study. It does not seem particularly helpful to do so since the tables have not been set up to text specific hypotheses but rather to offer a descriptive survey of developmental trends. Differences and correlations discussed in the text, however, are generally significant at acceptable levels. For example, let us take Table 2.5, which shows the correlation between anxiety signs in the AI test and MCT. We can distinguish both between strong MCT signs and other MCT signs and between the left column of AI signs (strong signs) and the two right columns. The G-index of agreement (Holley and Guilford, 1964) is 0.61 in the lower age groups and 0.56 in the higher ones (and the p-values for the fourfold contrasts < 0.005). Testing the left column of italicized figures in Table 2.8 against the sum of the two right columns yields a corrected χ^2_C of 3.91 ($df = 2$, $p < 0.10$, one-tailed). With the two lower rows added, a more correct procedure in this case, we obtain a Fisher's exact p of 0.028. This goes to show how easy it is to test individual trends in our data. But it would be misguided to let single p-values steer the discussion.

Many of the patterns exhibited in our tables do not need much discussion because they only confirm what most investigators in the field already agree on. It is not particularly earthshaking to assert that prepuberty is an age of firm emotional control rather than a period of low emotional tide. Nor is it astonishing to demonstrate that, as the child develops, egocentric defensive strategies are discarded for cognitively more mature ones. However, these more or less self-evident results do provide evidence for the applicability of PG methods to problems of anxiety and defense against anxiety (cf. Lindbom, 1968). Because of this, we believe that, other things being equal, our less obvious findings should also be seen as trustworthy.

A direct transfer of adult scoring principles to the present data would have made for the loss of much valuable information. To be sure, we have made a special effort to free ourselves from the conventional MCT and AI scoring routines. As a result, we have been able to define operationally several primitive defensive strategies. One of these is eye shutting by the hero, which seems closely related to what psychoanalysts term "denial." Another early but more persistent defensive tactic, hero duplication, has been noted before and taken to be clearly narcissistic. In his Defense Mechanism Test, Kragh (1969) refers signs of hero duplication to the defensive category "introjection: polymorphous identification," whereas Andersson and Weikert (1974) employ the term "projected introjection" to represent a constellation of hero-threat interpretations at least partly comparable to hero duplication. Nevertheless, the relation of hero duplication to classical psychoanalytic mechanisms remains obscure. We have thus avoided substituting a debatable reference to psychoanalytic concepts for direct reference to the concrete MCT data.

Of central importance is the description the present study provides of how the defensive strategies develop from age 7 to 15. In their discussion of psychoanalysis and learning theory, Sandler and Joffe (1968) claim that old structures are never entirely lost when new ones are acquired; they are simply inhibited. This assumption dovetails nicely with our finding that primitive defense mechanisms dominate the C-phase in young children but are shoved back to the P-phase in older children, as more mature mechanisms come to the fore. The complete disappearance of the primitive mechanisms in most of the older children, even in the P-phases, does not necessarily mean that the old structures have been obliterated. It might be that the PG series we employed was too brief to allow for a reconstruction of all the early stages.

The succession over age of various kinds of mechanisms is rather well illustrated by our data in spite of the limited size of the sample. Eye shutting by the hero remains an effective strategy only as long as the child is bound by an egocentric view of reality. A more mature child turns the head of the threatening A_2 instead of the head of the hero. The shift to this rather more compulsive type of mechanism, however, is not a direct one; it proceeds via the narcissistic strategy of hero duplication. Only when hero duplication becomes obsolete does turning away assert itself as a mechanism in its own right. To complicate matters, eye shutting by the hero and hero duplication seem to be retained in disguised form in many adults. The more developed forms of repression may not relate directly to the eye-shutting (denial) strategy practiced by the younger children, although reports of lifeless stiffness may imply a rather sophisticated denial of danger (not really effective until a subject has learned to differentiate between representational objects and reality). Yet one might well designate as "partial denial" such early forms of repression as the reporting of isolated parts of the hostile face. Moreover, as argued above, the primitive stereotypy found in immature adults may be a distant variant of hero duplication.

It is interesting, in this connection, to consider certain attempts by psychoanalysts to differentiate denial from other forms of defense, particularly from repression. Jacobson (1957), among others, claims to have made a clear distinction between the two. As Sjöbäck (1973) points out, however, most of Jacobson's observations are based on the case history of a single patient. Moreover, Jacobson's essential argument seems only to apply to denial directed against the outside world. Her attempts to differentiate between repression and denial do not seem convincing to Sjöbäck because "each characteristic of denial proposed by her seems to exclude some phenomena ascribed to the operation of that mechanism from being explained in terms of it" (pp. 227–228). Sjöbäck sensibly suggests that any "adequate definition of the denial mechanism . . . will require, it seems, to be in some way or other hierarchically ordered" (p. 231). The developmental aspect inherent in the PG method is by definition hierarchical. Our data undoubtedly facilitate not only a differentiation between early (primitive) and late (mature) mechanisms, but also a description of how the latter succeed the former and how remnants of early strategies are retained within a more mature defensive armor.

Two other discoveries remain to be discussed. One is the existence of so-called leaking mechanisms in children with symptoms of anxiety. Even if these children try to cope with anxiety with the same strategies normal children use, their attempts remain ineffective. It should also be noted that these children seem more reluctant than normals to abandon their childish mechanisms and turn, for example, to "ordinary" compulsive mechanisms. Paraphrasing Schur (1953), we might say that in these youngsters the more mature strategy cannot (yet) forestall a regression toward primary anxiety, with the concomitant, more primitive forms of defense. However, we leave further speculations on these matters to our more systematic study of child psychiatric patients in Part Two, where differences in cognitive maturity are taken into account.

A final discovery to be mentioned is the characteristic presence of retention in young (normal) children. These children retain old interpretations together with new ones where older children would discard them. Such a lack of elimination may be taken at the same time as a sign of open communication between early and late phases of percept genesis. Since there were hardly any cases of retention in clinical children (despite their relative cognitive immaturity), it seemed that premature elimination might lead to fixation and a reduction of developmental alternatives. Phrasing this in more popular terms one could say: without retention there is no creativity.

In discussing defense mechanisms, we have of necessity touched on the problem of anxiety. It is true that the AI signs selected on logical grounds to serve as anxiety criteria correlated well with the MCT anxiety signs. It is also true that the clinical group differed from the normal group in the expected direction. Nevertheless, we need to supplement the data presented here with more detailed data from well-defined clinical groups before really confronting the issues of anxiety and defense as reflected in percept genesis.

One finding, however, is worth emphasizing at this point: the difference between younger and older children with respect to fusion of the hero and the threat. In the younger children, where the distinction between self and other is often not fully established on a cognitive level, one of the most imminent dangers would seem to be loss of identity when faced with a threatening world (cf. Greenacre, 1967). Or, to rephrase this in the spirit of Schur (1953), fusion of the ego and the source of danger renders any controlled appraisal difficult and facilitates direct, automatic reactions of helplessness. In some cases, where the hero and the threat seem to merge, one might even talk about regression to a symbiotic level.

In many important respects, our findings do not differ appreciably from what is by now common knowledge in developmental psychology. But in some respects, we believe, our approach has contributed to an elucidation of new facets of anxiety. Our primary aim, however, is not to demonstrate that properly standardized instruments might serve as diagnostic tools among children and adolescents. Instead, our concern is to penetrate deeper into the terra incognita of the growing human being. What we hope to find are some of the factors determining which direction, whether toward a relative freedom from anxiety or toward a crippling by it, the developmental process will take.

3

SECOND STUDY OF
NORMAL PRESCHOOL CHILDREN

The central task of our second study was to examine manifestations of anxiety and defense against anxiety in children below school age (age 7 in Sweden). Here we tried to trace the precursors of adult defense mechanisms further back than we could in the first study.[1] Not only did we use the same tests as before, but we also selected young children with social backgrounds similar to those of the first group, allowing for comparisons. At the same time our investigation was meant to serve as a "normal" background for inquiries into manifestations of anxiety and defense in clearly maladapted and anxiety-ridden children.

SUBJECTS

There were 55 children in this second group of subjects, 25 boys and 30 girls. The youngest child was 3 years, 11 months, and the oldest one 6 years, 11 months. The children all came from two nursery schools located near the laboratory. Two children from these schools were not included: one boy with suspected brain lesion and another boy whose parents had already contacted the children's psychiatric clinic. Two 5-year-olds refused to continue after the tests had begun and two 4-year-olds did not want to participate at all. Undoubtedly, the time the experimenter took to acquaint herself with the children before bringing them to the laboratory was a factor in the low

[1] The lower age limit was determined by the minimum age for participation in the PG experiments (just below 4 years of age).

number of dropouts (see the section on Method).

Five children were under 5 years of age; 35 were between 5 years and 5 years, 11 months; and 15 were over age 6. (The proportion of boys to girls is dealt with below, in relation to the various subgroups.) While around 40% of the children in the first study came from well-educated families, the percentage was somewhat higher in this second group (45%).

The children were divided into groups according to age and cognitive maturity (as measured by the landscape test). In our first study, however, the cognitive test was more decisive in determining immature or mature groups. In this second study it was less strictly applied, as the age span was narrower.

Table 3.1 shows the breakdown of the age and cognitive maturity groups. The choice of one's own perspective in the landscape test is referred to as the X-choice and the selection of other perspectives as Y-choices. *Group 1* consists of all 4- and 5-year-olds who could not comprehend the landscape task at all, or failed to make the correct X-choice and made one or no correct Y-choice. This group is further divided into *subgroup 1a* (11 children not older than 5;6 with no comprehension) and *subgroup 1b* (the nine remaining children in group 1).

Group 2 includes all children 5;0 to 5;6 years of age with the correct X-choice and two or less correct Y-choices, all children 5;7 to 5;11 years with the correct X-choice but no correct Y-choices, and all 6-year-olds who failed to make the correct X-choice (most of them had two correct Y-choices). *Subgroup 2a* consists of 10 children 5;6 years or younger who made the correct X-choice and one or no correct Y-choice. *Subgroup 2b* includes the nine remaining children in group 2.

Group 3 includes all children 5;6 years or younger with all choices correct, the children 5;7 to 5;11 years with one or more correct Y-choice besides the correct X-choice, and all children 6 years or older with at least the correct X-choice. In *subgroup 3a* there are nine children with two or fewer correct Y-choices besides the correct X-choice. *Subgroup 3b* consists of the seven children with all choices correct.[2]

The proportion of boys to girls was fairly even in subgroups

---

[2] Certain comparison groups from the first study will be listed in some of the tables below. In these groups only Y-choice mistakes were scored.

TABLE 3.1
AGE AND COGNITIVE MATURITY LEVELS IN NORMAL PRESCHOOL GROUP

Landscape test	Age (years and months)			
	<5	5:0–6	5:7–11	6:0–11
No comprehension	*1a* 4	7	2	
Incorrect X* ± 1 correct Y	*1b* 1	3	3	1
Incorrect X + 2 correct Ys etc.	*2a*		*2b*	4
Correct X + 0 correct Ys		6	2	2
Correct X + 1 correct Y		*3a* 4	2	1
Correct X + 2 correct Ys	*2b*	2	1	3
Correct X + 3 correct Ys	*3b*	2	1	4

* X = choice of own perspective, Y = choice of other perspective.

1a (6:5), 1b (4:5), and 2a (5:5). In subgroup 2b there were two boys and seven girls, in subgroup 3a six boys and three girls, and in subgroup 3b two boys and five girls. The higher proportion of girls in subgroup 3b might have been expected.

METHOD

In Chapter 2 we mentioned some methodological problems specific to children as subjects in experimental research. These problems are intensified in a younger age group and new difficulties arise. The problem of diminished reliability in the younger age groups may at first seem insurmountable. Children below school age are not expected to endure a prolonged test or to understand and obey the test instructions. At the same time the experimenter has trouble understanding the child because of the child's very different use of language. Yet, despite these difficulties, we were able to ensure extended participation by our subjects. In addition to a critical evaluation of the children's verbal reports, we assessed the experimenter's observations of their behavior in the test situation.

As the first study indicates, the younger the child the more difficult it is to define a C-phase distinct from the preceding P-phases. In our youngest and most cognitively immature groups, many children never even identified the stimulus correctly. This observation may in itself be of interest. Without a stable C-phase, it becomes impossible to differentiate between latent and manifest contents or even between early and late PG segments. Thus, the manifestations of anxiety and defense in these young children have to be defined differently from those in older and more mature children. A key problem is how to conceptualize the experience of anxiety in subjects in whom the differentiation of an experiencing self (the P-phase part) from outside reality (the C-phase part) is not yet clearly established.

It was particularly important to prepare these children for the tests. The experimenter took time to become acquainted with them, often meeting with them several days beforehand. Once a kind of friendship was set up, it was generally not difficult to ensure the children's participation. The experimenter also tried to make the tests as pleasant as possible for the children. One result of these efforts was a surprisingly low loss of subjects.

In the first investigation with schoolchildren we paid special attention to problems of reliability. As noted above, these problems were expected to be exaggerated in a group of even younger children. For this reason, we devoted more time and care to the scoring of the MCT, particularly to the consideration of ambiguous and diffuse answers. Some of these problems will be discussed in presenting our results.

One possible difficulty is that, for the most part, our subjects cannot be expected to report everything they observe on the screen. Instead, they assume, as Piaget (1929) has pointed out, that the experimenter already knows what they are going to say. This was nicely illustrated by children just on the verge of leaving the egocentric stage, who somewhat doubtfully asked the experimenter whether she hadn't seen the same things. Such obstacles to full reporting can, to some extent, be overcome if the experimenter questions the child. When asking questions, however, the experimenter has to be very careful not to influence the child's answers.

As we have mentioned, young children are apt to express themselves nonverbally to a high degree. In order to maximize this kind of self-expression, the test rules were not stringently adhered to, but applied in a liberal and playful spirit. An anxious child, for example, might be allowed to sit on the experimenter's lap for a while, before continuing testing. Our choice was often between obtaining some relevant information or no information at all from the young child.

AFTERIMAGE TEST RESULTS

One reason for the inclusion of the AI test in our first study with schoolchildren was its diagnostic value, as shown by other investigations (Andersson, Nilsson, Ruuth, and Smith, 1972). Above all, signs of anxiety and of compulsive and hypersensitive reactions proved to be useful in characterizing certain age groups and differentiating normal and clinical children. Another reason for the use of this test was its known correlation with cognitive maturity or, generally speaking, with the observer's perspective on his own self in relation to the outside world. In our second study the latter reason becomes more prominent than the former: the AI data can be used to supplement the description furnished by the landscape test of the child's private epistemology.

As the reader may remember, the normal adult AI in our experiment would be negative (blue, blue-green), relatively dark compared with the bright schematic face, and larger than the stimulus (8.3 cm if exactly proportional to the projection distance, most often slightly larger). These characteristics of the AI purportedly reflect an operational perspective on the relation between self and outside physical reality, i.e., a mature understanding of the difference between a subjective product and the stable, objective environment. In this adult view of the AI, it is "projected by me" onto the outside world and hence apt to grow in proportion to the increased projection distance. Another sign of a clear differentiation between self and nonself is the negative color and low brightness.

A child who has not yet acquired the operational perspective but appraises the world exclusively from his own point of view is bound to produce positive (red, brownish, violet) AIs which remain constant in size (Ruuth and Smith, 1969; Smith and Sjöholm, 1970, 1971). For the egocentric child, there is no distinct difference between his own projections onto the outside world and the physical attributes of that world. Consequently, the AI is seen as a physical object among other objects and does not change its size relative to an object such as the projection screen when the screen is moved away from the subject. This explains the size constancy of the immature AI. The positive color common among egocentric children has been interpreted as another sign of their confusion of the AI phenomenon with the AI stimulus.

Even the egocentric child, however, has a stable-enough relation between self and world to allow him to produce an AI and to hold it for close scrutiny and measurement. Before he acquires an egocentric perspective, the child is apt to be more directly dependent on the momentary stimulus situation and to lack any clear definition of self as distinct from nonself. Characteristically, such a child does not even prefer his own perspective in the landscape test, as he cannot yet comprehend the meaning of "my own perspective." This immature child probably finds it difficult to place the AI phenomenon within his field of experience or to concentrate on it for any length of time.

In adult subjects, anxiety is reflected in AI data by large images (10–11 cm or more), very dark images (brightness estimates of 9, 10, or more), and sometimes also by positive color (regressive reactions). Although we used these signs in the study of schoolchildren, when a subject's estimates of size (or his color experience) were uncertain because his self-nonself relations were still tinged by cognitive immaturity, the presence of large AIs (or of positive hues) could not be interpreted as reflecting anxiety. With the younger children in the present study not only AI size and color but also AI brightness could not be scored for anxiety signs in most cases since few children could make brightness judgments. (Because of this, we must postpone a further discussion of our use of AI data to estimate anxiety until the clinical group has been presented.) Other AI signs, such as green color (a sign of compulsive defenses) or variegated images (a sign of sensitivity), might be useful even in young children, but these signs were too rare to be significant in our sample (see the right column in Table 3.2).

In Table 3.2 we have separated the results for subjects lacking a clear egocentric perspective (1a, 1b), subjects clearly beyond the egocentric stage (3b), and the bulk of egocentric children (2a, 3b, 3a). It is evident that the youngest and most immature subjects cannot hold AIs for inspection — AIs simply do not concern them. In the most immature group (1a), only one child was able to measure as many as eight images; one other could measure a few of them. All differences between group 1 and the other groups are highly significant under the Fisher's exact test for 2×2 contingency tables.

The egocentric middle groups are characterized by images constant in size (6.5 cm or less). In many cases, all the AIs were small. Even here contrasts are significant ($p < 0.0075$, Fisher's exact test, one-tailed, between subgroups 2a + 2b + 3a and group 7–10[11] immature in columns 4 and 5 in Table 3.2). As the "cracking" of the egocentric perspective continues, size constancy eventually disappears. There are no AI serials with all images constant in size in subgroup 3b or at higher age levels. Another sign of growing uncertainty in subgroups 2a, 2b, and 3a with respect to size relations is that seven of 22 subjects reported at least two AIs larger than 10.5 cm.

Positive colors, or an absence of negative ones, continue to a later age than size constancy. Reflections of such primitive stimulus dependence are often observed in puberty and older age groups, although the positive phases here are generally very few and concentrated in early sections of the serials, sections where "early" adaptive strategies are most likely to be apparent. With growing age and maturity, positive phases are more and more often interspersed with negative ones.

TABLE 3.2
AI Test Results in Preschool and School-Age Children

Group	No AIs	< 8 AIs*	Rest of sample	All AIs ≤ 6.5 cm	Rest of sample	≥ 2 AIs ≤ 6.5 cm	Rest of sample	Only positive ≠ achromatic AIs	Rest of sample	≥ 2 AIs positive	Rest of sample	No negative-chromatic AIs	Rest of sample	Green AI color	Rest of sample
4-6															
1a + 1b	14	2	4	1	3	4	0	2	2	2	2	4	0	0	4
2a + 2b + 3a	1	6	21	8	13	19	4	6	15	8	15	14	8	1	22
3b	1	0	6	0	6	6	0	2	4	2	4	4	2	0	6
7-10(11) immature	2	0	17	0	17	7	10	2	15	6	11	4	13	5	12
7-10(11) mature	0	1	16	0	16	3	14	1	15	9	7	4	12	5	11
(11)12-13	0	1	16	0	16	1	15	0	16	6	10	0	16	10	7
14-15	0	0	19	0	19	1	18	1	18	6	13	3	16	5	14

* We have used these incomplete AI serials in the other columns specifying AI size and color *only* if the data permitted a definite conclusion about the serial had it been complete. For instance, if a subject reported only three AIs, we could not consider him under the column "all AIs ≤6.5 cm." However, if two of his three AIs were ≤6.5 cm, he could be included in this column.

META-CONTRAST TECHNIQUE RESULTS

ANXIETY

In our investigation of schoolchildren we found a clear difference between signs of anxiety in subjects around or just before puberty and signs in younger subjects. We could hardly expect to transfer the scoring principles used for even the youngest of our schoolchildren to all age levels in the preschool group. One important characteristic of the subgroups with the youngest and most immature preschool children seems to be that they cannot yet clearly distinguish an inner world from an outer one. What we term "anxiety" in an adult or older child is primarily associated with the person's private self. In contrast, the younger and more cognitively immature the child, the more closely anxiety must be linked to the outside situation. It would, then, seem more appropriate to talk about fright (or *Realangst*) than about anxiety. Anxiety, in the true sense of the word, is internalized fright.

As we shall see in more detail in the next section, immature defensive strategies are often not represented in the children's perceptual reports per se but rather are disclosed in direct action. Here their attempts to flee or their search for comforting shelter with the experimenter can also be seen as typical signs of "anxiety." Somatic reactions belong to a similar category. It seems reasonable to assume that the test situation itself is more stressful for young children than for more experienced ones. Signs of fright and tension are therefore expected to be quite common. We need only mention the counterphobic manipulations so often encountered among our subjects—their wish to touch everything, to do it themselves, "to handle the very source of danger," as it were (compare also the active forgetting and distracting behavior noted below).

In spite of all this, we wish to trace those signs in the present group which correlated best with AI signs of anxiety among the younger schoolchildren: real zero-phases, hero discontinuity, and fusion. A *zero-phase* was scored when the subject reported seeing nothing, or nothing meaningful; *hero discontinuity,* when the hero (in B_2) was said to have disappeared; *fusion,* when the hero and the threat (or the interpretation representing A_2) were

TABLE 3.3
ANXIETY SIGNS IN MCT

Group	Zero-phases	Hero discontinuity	Fusion	Some of these 3 signs	None of these 3 signs	Fright
4-6						
1a	4	1	3	7 ⎫	4 ⎫	3
1b	3	2	1	4 ⎬ 11	5 ⎬ 9	2
2a	4	1	4	6 ⎫	4 ⎫	1
2b	2	4	1	5 ⎬ 11	4 ⎬ 8	1
3a	1	2	0	2 ⎫	7 ⎫	1
3b	1	1	2	3 ⎬ 5	4 ⎬ 11	1
7-10(11)				11	23	
(11)12-15				1	35	

mixed up or had close physical contact. Considering the expected risk of diminished reliability in lower age and maturity groups, especially with regard to signs of this type, we were extremely cautious in scoring them. A zero-phase was, for instance, not scored if an answer such as "I did not have time to see anything" might have been interpreted as inattention or unwillingness to report. Hero discontinuity was noted only in cases where the subject explicitly pointed to the absence of the hero (not when he merely failed to mention him). Similarly, fusion was not recorded when the mix-up might have derived from the experimenter's inability to fully understand the subject's description of his percept.

Zero-phases were scored in 15 cases and hero discontinuity and fusion in 11 cases each. Comparing the relative frequencies of this material with the 7-10(11)-year-olds of Study 1, we found about the same frequency in the preschool group 3 but much higher ones in the other groups (Table 3.3). In addition, reports of A_2 as something frightening were scored in nine cases here, five of them in group 1. Direct expressions of fright (in the subject himself or in the hero) were not identified with certainty in any of the schoolchildren.

Since the misperception of A_2 often represents a defense against the threat, disintegration of such perceptual formations may well be a sign of incipient anxiety. Yet even in our study of schoolchildren, we found that such *structural disintegration* was not necessarily an indication of anxiety in the younger members of the group as their perceptual reports were rather unstable anyway. Medium strong anxiety signs in the younger schoolchildren, such as *broken structures* ("a cracked window-pane"), or *phobic formations* (objects), were relatively rare in the preschool group. On the other hand, *dark structures* that did not correspond to dark areas in the stimulus — another medium strong sign — were scored in 10 children, evenly distributed over all subgroups.

As we have noted above, no AIs were produced by many of the youngest and most immature children; other children could not estimate the AI intensity. In the first study, we decided not to regard large AIs as indicative of anxiety if size-constant AIs were also reported in the same series. The reason was that the enlarged AI in such cases might simply be a sign of the subject's general (cognitive) uncertainty about the "position" of a visual AI in his world of experience, and not an unequivocal sign of anxiety. Because of these ambiguities, we cannot validate the postulated MCT signs of anxiety by using AI data. The final judgment of the MCT as an instrument for assessing anxiety in very young children must await the test results of children with clear clinical symptoms of anxiety.

Nevertheless, we would like to consider here the accumulation of zero-phases, hero discontinuity, and fusion in the youngest and most immature groups. The reader might expect some correlation between such signs and the greater inability of young children to report a stable and unambiguous meaning of B (in the introductory and control series). Eight children in subgroup 1a were scored for "subjectivity" in the C-phase (Series 1 or Series 2 or both) compared with only three children altogether in subgroups 3a and 3b. This skewed age distribution, however, does not necessarily signify that the signs of anxiety discussed here directly correlate with the lack of an unambiguous C-phase. In fact, the G-coefficient of agreement (Holley and Guilford, 1964) between these two sets of data only reaches the insignificant value of 0.13.

The anxiety signs just discussed did prove to be meaningful

in early school-age children who, according to their test results, were still marked by an egocentric perspective but who, within the bounds of such a perspective, had probably started to draw a line between the inside and outside aspects of their experiential world. For these children, any break in the stability of this construction must be felt as threatening. The same is also true, we believe, of the older children among our preschoolers, above all group 3. The more diffuse the difference between self and nonself in the child's world of experience, the more frequently one can expect such signs of instability and fusion and, possibly, the less indicative they are of anxiety. As noted above, however, younger children may be more frightened by the test situation than older ones so that the accumulation of reports of instability and fusion at lower age levels may, to some extent at least, reflect a real state of anxiety.

PRIMITIVE MECHANISMS

The child psychologist, or the observant parent for that matter, might well expect to find two types of defense in the youngest and most immature children: direct denial of the threatening reality or attempts to flee from it. These averting strategies appear not only, or even primarily, on the perceptual level, but also on the behavioral level. That is, they are found not so much in what the child reports about the MCT picture but in how he acts in the testing situation.

Direct denial includes *eye-shutting behavior* (the child shuts his own eyes or otherwise avoids looking at the screen), *sleep behavior* (similar to eye-shutting behavior but accompanied by talk about sleepiness or tiredness, yawning, etc.), and *no C-phase* (when the child refuses to identify A_2, even at the longest possible exposure time).

Direct flight or *shelter-seeking behavior* refers to attempts by the subject to escape from the situation by walking away, for instance, or by cuddling next to the experimenter. We shall distinguish between flight and seeking shelter in our scoring. Thus, when flight is cited in the tables, we do not mean seeking shelter unless this is explicitly stated.

Flight behavior is considered the most primitive defensive

strategy and is typical of children who are still relatively close to the sensorimotor stage (as defined by Piaget). Eye-shutting behavior seems to require a more established egocentric perspective, in which self and nonself can be distinguished as separate poles in the child's field of experience. However, although the child using the eye-shutting strategy is capable of denying outside reality, he is not yet capable of differentiating between a real object and the representation of that object. He thus cannot transfer his defensive strategy to the pictorial level. It does not help the child to see the MCT hero as shutting his eyes, the child has to shut his own.

Table 3.4 shows very clearly that in the youngest and most immature children (subgroup 1a) — those who cannot yet understand the landscape task or find a place for the AI phenomenon in their world of experience — the dominant strategy is one of direct flight. Eye-shutting behavior appears somewhat later. Flight and shelter-seeking behavior are also more typical of subgroups 1a and 1b than of the other ones. If we combine flight and eye-shutting behavior, the difference between subgroups 1a and 3b becomes total ($p \ll 0.001$, Fisher's exact test, two-tailed). (Remember that subgroup 3b is made up of older children who have accepted a concrete-operational perspective, i.e., who manage to solve the entire landscape test and also to produce reasonably mature AIs.)

A number of other reactions seem to follow a similar distribution curve, e.g., *motor unrest,* or an inability to sit reasonably still, and *somatic manifestations,* such as a sudden craving for food or water, an urgent need to go to the bathroom, etc. What is interesting about these behaviors is that they usually do not appear until the threatening A_2 has been introduced at a subliminal level.

Two types of reactions less clearly related to age and cognitive maturity are *forgetting* (the child pretends to have forgotten what he just saw and says that he did not have enough time to look properly or gives similar evasive answers) and *distracting behavior* (the child maneuvers to shift the conversation to less dangerous topics). Compared with the other reactions, these two strategies seem to imply attempts at active mastery of the situation.

Another defensive category, which should be described in

TABLE 3.4

PRIMITIVE AND RELATED (NARCISSISTIC) STRATEGIES IN MCT

Group	Direct denial (number of times scored) ≥2	1	0	Flight-shelter (number of times scored) 2	1	0	Only flight behavior	Flight + eye shutting	Eye shutting and/or doubtful flight behavior	Only eye shutting	Rest of sample	Flight and/or eye shutting	Rest of sample	Motor unrest +	−	Somatic manifestations +	−	Forgetting +	−	Distracting behavior +	−	Primitive isolation +	−	Hero duplication, eye shutting by hero, etc* +	−
4–6																										
1a	5	3	3	6	4	1	7	3	1	0	0	11	0	4	7	4	7	4	7	7	4	6	5	2(1)	9(10)
1b	4	2	3	1	4	4	1	2	9	1	6	4	5	3	6	0	9	4	5	5	4	2	7	7(6)	2(3)
2a	3	4	3	0	3	7						3	7	7	3	2	8	1	9	4	6	2	8	8(6)	2(4)
2b	2	2	5	1	1	7	1	1	10	1	5	5	4	3	6	0	9	2	7	4	5	2	7	3(1)	6(8)
3a	2	3	4	1	1	7	1	1	0	1	2	3	6	3	6	0	9	1	8	3	6	0	9	4(3)	5(6)
3b	0⁻	1	6	0	1	6	0	0	1	2	4	0	7	1	6	1	6	2	5	4	3	0	7	4(3)	3(4)
7–8 immature	Not seen			Not seen										Not scored		Not scored		Not scored		Not scored		Not seen		9(6)	0(3)
7–8 mature																								2(1)	5(6)
9–10(11) immature																								6(2)	4(8)
9–10(11) mature																								3(0)	7(10)

* Figures within parentheses refer to cases where these defenses were scored more than once and immediately before the termination of the series.

connection with flight and eye-shutting behavior, involves overt actions vis-à-vis the stimulus picture. Certain children were very eager to walk up to the screen or to move their chair forward in order to scrutinize the picture close up, particularly the area around the window in B_2. We see this behavior partly as an attempt to isolate the threatening image from the rest of the picture (an intention often indicated by the child's gestures), and partly as a kind of weapon — overpowering and controlling the threat by persistent staring. We have called this strategy *primitive isolation.* It was scored most often in subgroup 1a and was never noted among normal children 7 years of age or older. The relation between primitive isolation, on the one hand, and compulsive isolation in older children, on the other, will be discussed in the section below on magical and compulsive strategies.

In the study of schoolchildren (Chapter 2), a strategy called *primitive repression* was identified, characterized by the child's mentioning only single, detached parts of A_2 (a strand of hair, an ear, a nose, etc.). This particular defense will be treated later, together with other repressive signs. Compared with primitive isolation, it seems to be a relatively advanced form of defense, on a par with shutting the hero's eyes or hero duplication (which will now be discussed).

As soon as the child has learned to distinguish between an object and its representation, the prerequisites exist for defensive manipulations of the *picture* instead of direct action in the "real world." An important consequence is an increase in the possibilities for differentiating defensive strategies. First of all, the subject may substitute *eye shutting and shelter seeking by the hero* for his own behavior. Among the older children, eye shutting by the hero was often associated with *hero duplication,* a narcissistic strategy where a duplicate of the hero is placed in the window instead of the threatening face. Whether we consider the general frequency of such strategies or only cases where they dominate the C-phase (see Table 3.4), there is no clearly significant peak of these signs among the preschoolers, although they seem to be most frequent in subgroups 1b and 2a. We can say, however, that eye shutting by the hero and hero duplication are more typical of an older age than flight and eye-shutting behavior. In the immature 7- to 8-year-olds, for instance, eye shutting by the hero and hero duplication were quite common, whereas flight and eye-shutting behavior were not noted at all.[3] Yet, although it is a more advanced tactic, the effectiveness of eye shutting by the hero as a defense depends on the degree to which an egocentric perspective still governs the child's reasoning. The same can be said of hero duplication. With increasing age and loosening ego-centrism, this strategy no longer dominates the C-phase, although it still appears sporadically at a P-phase level in older and more mature children, as well as in adults (see Chapter 2).

PROJECTIVE STRATEGIES

The most typical sign of projection in the MCT, at least the sign which best illustrates the "mechanics" behind hypersensitive and paranoid attributions, is a *change in the perception of B influenced by the subliminal perception of A,* i.e., the subject does not identify A directly but via a detour in the established B percept. (The control series is used here as the base level for judging what should be regarded as a change in B influenced by A.) Other signs of projection have been defined through validation work with adult subjects. Drastic B-changes, such as the addition of live crea-tures or breaks in the phase-to-phase continuity, have been scored even after A has been sensed within B. Identification of A_2 or the hero as intimate associates of the subject (e.g., father, mother, psychiatrist), interaction between the hero and A_2 (e.g., exchange of meaningful glances), movement, etc., are other scoring categories that have proved valid in identifying hyper-sensitive and paranoid individuals. These categories were used in our study of schoolchildren.

Table 3.5 shows the distribution of the MCT signs of projec-tion in our second study. Eighteen children reported the appear-ance of *extra human beings or animals in B* after Series 1 or 2 had reached the section of double exposures. Eight additional child-ren did not show this sign but reported *other drastic changes in B,* such as a transformation of the interior in Series 1 into a land-

---

[3] In ongoing work, where we have looked specifically for these signs in the 7- to 8-year-olds, we *have* found them, but their incidence was much lower than in the preschool children.

TABLE 3.5
SIGNS OF PROJECTION IN MCT*

Group	X_1	X_2	Y	Z
1a	5	2	0	4
1b	0 ⎤	2 ⎤	2 ⎤	5 ⎤
2a	3 ⎦ 3	4 ⎦ 6	1 ⎦ 3	2 ⎦ 7
2b	3 ⎤	1 ⎤	0 ⎤	5 ⎤
3a	1 ⎦ 4	4 ⎦ 5	3 ⎦ 3	1 ⎦ 6
3b	0	1	1	5

*X   = Extra persons/animals or other drastic B-change in A + B section.
X_1 = X with B not attaining C-phase level.
X_2 = X with B attaining C-phase level.
Y   = The rest with less drastic signs (i.e., not including those who also showed X signs).
Z   = The rest without signs.

scape with roads. Perceptions of A_2 *or the hero as a familiar person* and reports of interaction between the threat and the hero were only found in a few cases. *Subtle B-changes* (where the phase-to-phase continuity of B was not endangered by shifts, for instance, in the perspective or lighting of the room) were scored in seven cases, and *activity by the hero or the threat* or other kinds of movement in 12 cases. These last, "less drastic" signs of projection were tallied together (in Table 3.5, however, column Y represents only those children with less drastic signs who did *not* also show X signs).

Since many of the preschool children did not attain the C-phase level for B when this stimulus was presented alone (i.e., before the A + B section), we decided to differentiate the drastic projection signs accordingly. In other words, we distinguished between (1) drastic signs in children without a C-phase for B and (2) drastic signs in children with a clear C-phase (see Table 3.5). The C-phase is here defined as a correct description of the major visual structures in B, free from subjective distortions (except for minor details) and not changed or lost in the control series. Among the subjects with less drastic signs of projection, a C-phase was lacking in only one case. Thus, no differentiation with respect to C-phase was used.

As long as the child does not report a stable, objective C-phase, B-changes do not suggest much more than a corroboration of total P-phase dominance in the PG process. Following

Anna Freud (1936), we hesitate to use the term "projection" when there is still no clear indication of a differentiation between the source of projection and its outside object (cf. Freud's [1920] distinction between projection proper and its precursors). As soon as an "independent" perspective is established by the child, however, the concept of projection becomes meaningful. Certainly, very drastic changes in B imply a lack of fundamental constancy in the child's conception of the world. Nevertheless, once the child can report a stable C-phase, these signs should be considered in light of their projective aspects.

Although the differences between the various subgroups just fail to reach the 0.05 level of significance, the trend in Table 3.5 seems convincing. P-phase dominance is most pronounced in subgroup 1a (the youngest children, who do not yet have even an egocentric perspective). P-phase dominance has completely vanished in subgroup 3b, where cognitive egocentrism is definitely passé. In the middle subgroups real projection is substituted for primitive P-phase dominance. Drastic signs are mixed with less drastic variants; in many cases only the latter were scored. It should also be mentioned that in the first study drastic signs were almost never recorded among the schoolchildren. Furthermore, when such signs are found in adults, they automatically lead one to suspect paranoia.

Here we particularly wish to emphasize the simultaneous presence at the egocentric stage of (1) an established and, in a superficial sense at least, objective C-phase and (2) very pronounced projective mechanisms. In our view, the children in subgroups 1b–3a build their image of the outside world from within themselves; that is, they provide their own substance and meaning to what they see, to the point of fabricating additional human beings and animals, even though they are now aware of certain constant perceptual facts. We can thus trace the development of our 4- to 6-year-olds from a stage of accidental dependencies (where outer referents cannot be clearly separated from inner ones) to a stage of subjective expansion with progressively more established realistic contours. On the other side of this expansive period, we glimpse a third phase, more deeply rooted in a reality common to all observers.

In many ways this description seems quite close to Piaget's

description of cognitive development from the late sensorimotor phase, through the egocentric phase, to the concrete-operational phase (see Piaget, 1926; Piaget and Inhelder, 1966). The major difference would be that in our study this developmental progression is not illustrated exclusively on a cognitive level. Our data reflect reactions to threatening or aversive stimuli — emotional processes of anxiety and defense against anxiety. These processes are of course related to the subject's degree of cognitive maturity. The close association to Piaget's findings can probably be taken as a substantiation of our assumption that projective strategies fill not only a defensive role in the child's life but also, to a considerable degree, an adaptive function. They are a means to the child's successful construction of reality.

MAGICAL AND COMPULSIVE STRATEGIES

The most common compulsive response in our first study of schoolchildren was *turning away the head of the threat,* i.e., the child saw A_2 from behind instead of *en face.* In the youngest and most immature schoolchildren such responses were often combined with hero duplication (see the discussion of primitive mechanisms). Other useful categories borrowed from the MCT manual for adults were *isolation* (e.g., a white surface instead of A_2 or curtains covering the window in B_2), *negation* ("anyhow, it's *not* an angry man"), *empty serials* (where the reports of B_2 remain unchanged and A_2 is not noted until it can be correctly identified), and *empty faces* (when the subject perceives an empty oval without features or expression instead of a face in the window). Two additional response categories were regarded as closely related to compulsion: *perceptual manipulation* and *intellectualization.* As noted in Chapter 2, in the first type of response the subject concentrates on details, often around the window in B_2; in the second type the threat is transported to the realm of mere thought or imagination.

In the first study the "golden age" for all sorts of compulsive strategies, as evidenced in the AI test as well as the MCT, was prepuberty (12–13 years). At the age levels adjacent to our second group of children (7–8 years), compulsive responses were much less frequent. Even turning away the head was relatively uncommon, and, as just noted, it was scored mostly in combination with hero duplication. For this reason, we expected a relatively low showing of compulsive strategies in the preschool group. Turning away the head was scored twice, empty faces twice (and reluctantly), isolation three times, intellectualization four times, negation five times, completely empty serials six times, and perceptual manipulation six times (in a total of 21 children). Five additional cases of *isolationlike* reports could be counted. Another category, *belittling* ("it's only a small one in the window"), was scored only three times. *Cleavage,* or temporal differentiation of A and B long before any C-phase, may be considered as related to the compulsive strategies; this response had the greatest frequency (10 cases).

In looking for primitive defenses, we also noted a kind of *primitive isolation* in some children's attempts to subjugate or control the threat directly at close range. This mechanism was particularly common among the youngest and most immature subjects. The magical components in this kind of defense are only too obvious. The same is partly true of other primitive defenses such as eye-shutting behavior and forgetting, where the child tries to escape the threat by undoing what has happened. Even the absence of a C-phase in a child's protocol may reflect a magical attempt to dismiss the threat by not recognizing or naming it. As a matter of fact, among the 22 subjects who did not report A_2, nine made an ugly face themselves toward the end of the test.

Considering the central role magic is supposed to play in the compulsive patterns of defense, we decided to take stock of other forms of magical behavior in the MCT situation. We found children, for instance, who used stylized strings of words before an exposure, or seemingly omnipotent children, who ordered the threat to recede or the MCT apparatus to stop functioning. Some formalized finger or mouth games also appeared to belong to this primitive category of magic rituals. A more abstract way of gaining control over the situation was counting the number of exposures. Another sophisticated pattern of magical control was seen when the child denied taking part in the test by keeping his coat on during the entire test or by speaking in a self-effacing, whispering voice. These latter forms of denial, together with counting, are regarded here as closer to adult forms of compulsion than sorcery and games.

The trends in Table 3.6 are not completely clear except insofar as primitive isolation is concerned. Here the difference between subgroup 1a and group 3, for instance, is highly significant ($p = 0.0032$, Fisher's exact test, two-tailed). Moreover, the more primitive forms of magical behavior tend to cluster in the low-level groups and the more complicated forms in the higher ones. The compulsionlike categories of perceptual manipulation, cleavage, and intellectualization are also more common in the middle and oldest groups. True compulsive strategies, as has already been pointed out, do not develop until much later.

Although there are no clear signs of compulsive defenses in children before prepuberty, we might cautiously link primitive isolation and magic rituals with adult compulsive strategies. Eye-shutting behavior and, to some extent, forgetting might also be seen as possible precursors of adult isolation and negation. The best indication that these early types of behavior resemble compulsion is their double character of sorcery and control. For instance, like compulsive adults, children using primitive isolation do not flee from the threat, do not "turn their backs to it," but rather try to neutralize it through rational-magical means (see the discussion of repressive strategies below). After the test some of these children were particularly meticulous in their drawings,[4] often making all the teeth in a big open mouth clearly visible.

Repressive Strategies

A common perceptual defense in adult hysterics and phobics is to convert the threat into a lifeless bust or mask or into a tree or some object. Since the threatening percept is drained of all human life, or "decathected," we have called this defensive tactic *repression*. Stimulus-near interpretations are most common in primitive hysterics and appear to contain elements of childish denial: "a lifeless mask can't be dangerous," "it's only a dressed-up theater actor," etc. Thoroughly "revised" versions of the

---

[4] Some children wanted to make drawings after the testing and they were encouraged to do so.

TABLE 3.6
MAGICAL AND COMPULSIVE MECHANISMS IN MCT

Group	Primitive isolation		Magic— more primitive forms		Magic— more advanced forms		Perceptual manipulation		Cleavage		Intellectual- ization	
	+	−	+	−	+	−	+	−	+	−	+	−
1a	6	5	6	5	0	11	0	11	0	11	0	11
1b	2	7	4	5	0	9	0	9	1	8	0	9
2a	2	8	3	7	1	9	1	9	3	7	1	9
2b	2	7	3	6	2	7	2	7	3	6	0	9
3a	0	9	3	6	4	5	1	8	2	7	2	7
3b	0	7	2	5	1	6	2	5	1	6	1	6

threat such as inanimate objects (a building, a radio, a bike) are more typical of anxiety hysterics and phobics.

Obviously the effectiveness of the stimulus-near type of repression depends on the subject's conceiving this artificial or theatrical world as being entirely different from the real world. As we well know, such a distinction is probably not possible for young children, so that the adult form of repression would be inefficient. As a matter of fact, we did not find a single case of stimulus-near repression in the immature 7- to 8-year-olds in the first study. Yet there were many instances of so-called *primitive repression* (A_2 was dismembered and described as a strand of hair, a nose, or half a face). Thus mutilated, A_2 no longer constituted a real threat.

Similarly, in this second study, we found virtually no stimulus-near repression. One case occurred in subgroup 2a. We did, however, note three instances of ostensibly repressive threat transformation. The threat was converted into a mask, a mountain, or a row of icicles; yet this did not alleviate the child's dread. Instead, the child expressed genuine alarm at this perception.

Reports classified as primitive repression seem more common, but we should note the difficulty in scoring this in some children. If the child talks about a head but emphasizes that the ears are white, this does not really mean that the child is reporting "torn-off" body parts. He saw the whole head to begin with. Using a very conservative scoring system, we marked nine cases of primitive repression — with greater latitude we could score another four. Only one case came from subgroup 1a; five cases were from subgroup 2a. In addition, two instances of animal substitutions were found, five reports of a tree, and three cases where A_2 was seen as an object. None of these children belonged to subgroup 1a.

In discussing primitive repression in our first study, we tentatively assumed a closer relation to partial denial than is the case with more adult types of repression. As we move down the age and maturity scale, even the primitive variants tend to disappear. Instead, direct denial or, at the lowest level, flight becomes a typical defensive strategy. We have just linked compulsive isolation to primitive isolation and magic. We would be even more justified in connecting repression with flight behavior (including eye-shutting behavior and forgetting). As we see it, the developmental chain is from direct flight to eye-shutting behavior or forgetting to partial denial or primitive repression and then to adult repression. In any case, adult repression, as scored in the MCT, has no direct counterpart in these young children but has to be considered a relatively late product of development.

OTHER TACTICS

In the first sample of schoolchildren, *retention* was scored when a child reported a new interpretation in phase N but at the same time retained the interpretation given in phase N − 1, thus balancing two or more meanings against each other. No case of retention was identified in our second sample. Possible reasons for this absence of retention will be presented at the end of the general discussion.

We also noted *leaking mechanisms* when indications of defensive formations and signs of anxiety occurred at the same time. These co-occurrences were particularly common in the clinical children, in whom the anxiety was most often combined with repression or isolation. Since, however, clear cases of mature repression and isolation were quite rare in the preschool group, we would not expect to find leaking mechanisms very often at this age level. Although simultaneous occurrences of anxiety and other defensive strategies were spotted here, we prefer to postpone the presentation of these to a comparison with clinical cases.

Since *transitional objects* (Winnicott, 1953) are reportedly quite common in preschoolers, one might have expected their projection onto the B_2 picture. Yet reports that the hero had a teddy bear or some other transitional object were surprisingly rare (only six cases).

Sex change in the hero was scored nine times, most often among the older children. Eight of these cases occurred in the older half of the group (age 5 ½ or above; $p = 0.020$, binomial test). One reason for this uneven distribution may be the younger children's lack of ability to identify with the hero (see our general discussion).

TRENDS OVER AGE: AN OVERVIEW

In viewing the main trends over age, we can distinguish three stages in the young children. Stage 1 refers to subgroup 1a; stage 2 to subgroups 2a and 2b; and stage 3 to subgroup 3b. Subgroups 1b and 3a should be considered transitional stages which sometimes reflect characteristics of the stage before, sometimes of the stage after (see Figure 3.1).

STAGE 1

The youngest and cognitively most immature children are still dominated by a direct sensorimotor relation to the world around them. "My own self" is not clearly distinguished from persons or objects out there. In other words, these children cannot yet differentiate object representations from objects, imagery from outside reality.

The landscape test thus seems totally irrelevant to these children. Even in choosing a photo from their own perspective, they pick the wrong one because all the photos are alike to them. Since the field of experience is dominated by immediate stimulus dependence, AIs are naturally difficult to comprehend and retain for inspection. It seems almost impossible to require children at this stage to shift their attention from the real stimulus object to its "subjective" aftereffect.

In the MCT, the children's reports may be both close to the stimulus and blatantly subjective at the same time. A well-defined C-phase of the B-stimulus, free from P-phase influence, is usually lacking. Defensive strategies are direct and open, involving tendencies to flee from the situation or attempts not to see the threat. But they are also marked by magical elements, including "concrete" isolation and control of the threat at close range.

It is assumed that at this stage children's anxiety is closely tied to the threatening situation and should therefore preferably be

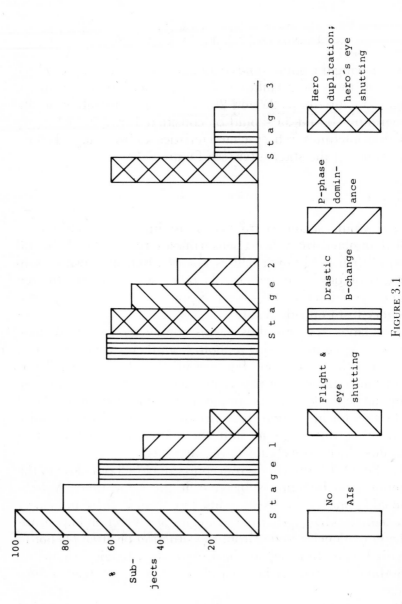

FIGURE 3.1

SCHEMATIC ILLUSTRATION OF THE CHANGE OVER AGE AND COGNITIVE MATURITY LEVELS OF SOME RESPONSE CATEGORIES.

called *Realangst* or fright. Here we encounter most of the open expressions of dread of A_2.

STAGE 2

This middle stage includes children who understand the landscape task but let choices of their own perspective dominate. The beginning differentiation of self and nonself is still mainly egocentric, i.e., they do not comprehend a world independent of themselves. This is reflected in AI data both by their ability to produce AIs and retain them for measurement and by the general size constancy of these images. What is produced by "me" becomes real, "out there."

Children at stage 2 are at first able to report a correct C-phase but, once the subliminal A is introduced, they often fill it with their own "live" content. The meaning of reality is primarily projected from within themselves. Moreover, remnants of primitive defense mechanisms are apparent. Beginning internalization is reflected in an increasing shift of early defensive tactics to the picture level, above all to the hero himself. The child no longer reacts simply to a direct threat coming from the outside but transports the whole problem into the world of representations. These internalized defenses, however, have a clearly narcissistic character (hero duplication, etc.). What is new is that the fear of outside danger typical of stage 1 now has an inner dimension, a reference to the child's own self. A transition to true anxiety has been made.

STAGE 3

The egocentric perspective no longer dominates at this stage. The children in group 3b can already master concrete-operational problems. Accordingly, even if still marked by primitive signs, their AIs swiftly lose their size constancy and begin to change size in proportion to the projection distance.

In the MCT the flow of projection peters out and the C-phase becomes more clearly established. Internalized defenses against "feelings" of danger and uneasiness have now been almost entirely substituted for direct warding off of an outside threat.

Even the narcissistic mechanisms of shutting the hero's eyes and hero duplication are no longer so dominant. Primitive repression, intellectualization, and perceptual manipulation can now be found. The lingering magical defenses become more and more ritualized and complicated.

DISCUSSION

Problems of reliability concerned us very much in the first study of schoolchildren and should, naturally, concern us still more in this second study of nursery school children.[5] Several precautions have thus been taken to check for uncontrolled variables. In the section on method, we noted that because of the children's inability to describe complicated impressions, their egocentric assumption that the experimenter already knew what they were thinking about, or their magical belief in not talking aloud about dangerous things, many of their reports were probably stripped of much important information. For instance, of the 12 children who grimaced at the end of Series 2 in the MCT (a sign of "identifying" perception as defined by Fenichel [1946]), nine did not report a correct A_2 (the grimacing face). We have also already indicated that by encouraging the child and only gently enforcing the test rules, the experimenter may have influenced the reports. The first problem cannot be ignored. Verbal reports, however, were only part of our data; nonverbal behavior became increasingly important with decreasing age. Moreover, we considered only what the child in fact reported, not the gaps and omissions in his reports. As far as the experimenter's influence is concerned, we should point out that if the children were unduly affected by the experimenter, which we very much doubt, the effect was certainly not systematic, nor was it favorable to our research hypotheses.

Even if we did succeed in measuring "something" in a fairly reliable way, how can we be sure that our data reflect anxiety and defense against anxiety? The differences between age and cognitive maturity groups recorded here may perhaps reflect an entirely different phenomenon, such as the development of

[5] The data presented for the preschool children have now been cross-validated (Smith and Carlsson, 1980).

ways of using insufficient information or ways of behaving when utterly bored (the latter is rather improbable since the behavior most closely related to boredom—distracting behavior—does not correlate with age or cognitive maturity). One indisputable fact is that the results from this study differ in many respects from our previous findings. Yet the data from schoolchildren also differed considerably from what we had encountered in adults, and they made sense only if we interpreted them as signs of how children try to master anxiety-provoking situations. Another fact in our favor is that, as in adults and schoolchildren, only the second MCT series seems to provoke defensive behavior; the first one reflects more of the subject's general perceptual "style." Since we presume that the test situation itself is more anxiety-provoking for the young child than for the older one, we feel all the more entitled to talk about anxiety and defense in interpreting our data. As noted above, the main problem is rather that in these youngsters many important manifestations, not so much of anxiety as of attempts to cope with it, have probably eluded our instruments.

In emphasizing the defensive aspects of our subjects' behavior, we may incur criticism for assigning common, apparently normal types of behavior to this "clinical" category. Yet a defensive arsenal is indispensable to every human being. In pointing to the obvious elements of defense in the coping strategies scored here, we should note that no clear dividing line can be drawn between defensive and adaptive strategies (cf. Hartmann's [1939] assumption that defense mechanisms originate in functions serving purely adaptive purposes). In the case of projection, for instance, the flooding of percepts with subjective content also seems to play a decisive part in the child's developing construction of reality; we thus agree with Novick and Kelly (1970) that "externalization" might be better than "projection" as a general term for processes leading to subjective allocation of internal phenomena to the external world. Primitive isolation may also serve an adaptive function: by first fixating and isolating the threat at close range, the child can then develop more systematic, general coping strategies. As we move to our investigation of clinical children (Part Two), however, we are more and more likely to meet strategies where the defensive aspect dominates at the expense of the adaptive one. In broad terms, such tactics often seem not only *non*adaptive but *mal*adaptive; to paraphrase Anna Freud (1965), they reflect the asymmetry along various developmental lines typical of the disturbed child. Ironically, with the growing prominence of its defensive aspect, a particular strategy often becomes less effective in dealing with the threat, at least in the long run.

As the MCT is a projective technique, a basic premise of its construction is that the subject's experiential world will be mirrored in his perceptions of the stimulus. We have learned, however, that an identification with the hero in Series 2 does not occur until the subject knows how to internalize his perceptions. In children who have not reached that stage, as our data show, the MCT does not serve as a true projective test; rather, it is a situational test, in which direct reactions to the stimuli are more characteristic of the subject than reports of his perceptions. Only gradually does dread of outside things change into an experience of dread "within me." One consequence of this transformation is that it is no longer sufficient for the child to deny outside danger; it becomes even more important to deny the apprehension of danger. This new perspective engenders more varied defensive manipulations. With abating egocentricity, adult forms of defense supersede childish ones.[6]

Before we have looked closely at anxiety-ridden children, it is not possible to state anything definite about manifestations of anxiety at different age levels. The AI test constitutes a special problem in this respect because the youngest children could not even produce AIs. In the MCT as well, judging from what we have just said about identification, we could expect visual representations of anxiety to be rather meager in subgroup 1a. In light of this, certain primitive defensive strategies were also seen as signs of anxiety. If flight or denial cannot be used as a means of escape, for instance, we will probably find direct expressions of dread or somatic reactions in these youngsters. Although visual anxiety manifestations increase with the beginnings

[6] Although in the MCT we have focused on reactions to the presence of aversive stimulation, we agree with Bowlby that "We are frightened not only by the *presence,* or expected presence, of situations of certain sorts, but by the *absence,* or expected absence, of *situations of other sorts*" (1973, p. 78; last italics ours).

of internalization, this does not mean that the scoring principles used for schoolchildren can be applied to the oldest and most mature nursery school children without thematic revisions. Even such strong signs of anxiety as fusion of the hero and the threat appear to have a different meaning in different age and cognitive maturity groups, probably partly because identity problems change as children pass into and out of the oedipal phase.

In trying to assess whether we have succeeded in discovering precursors of adult defense mechanisms and in tracing their development, we must reflect on the difficulties in drawing conclusions about developmental trends from a cross-sectional study. The problem becomes all the more complicated because the time interval between possible precursors and the full-fledged adult defenses may be considerable, as in the case of compulsive strategies. We have already discussed the successive internalization of defense. Here we would specifically like to examine the roots of such common defensive strategies as those found in hysterics and compulsives.

We have already postulated that compulsive isolation can be traced back to the primitive isolation of immature children, i.e., to their concrete isolation and control of the threat by "magic." If these tactics become ritualized and intellectualized, they may well form a bridge to the complicated rituals of adult compulsives or to the emotional isolation and intellectualization found in many normal adults. We are reminded here of Freud's (1915) speculation that compulsive defenses, like repression, are ultimately based on flight, but flight with unaverted eyes (see also Eissler, 1959). Our subjects with primitive isolation also try to see the danger.

We agree with most psychoanalysts that adult repression seems closely related to denial (see the discussion in Sjöbäck, 1973), and even to the "direct denial" found in our most immature children. Let us add here in passing that Spitz (1961) pointed to eye shutting as early as the very first year of life and called it a "prototype" of denial. Our young children's reports of torn-off body parts could be interpreted as both primitive repression and partial denial (of the threatening stimulus). We also often found a kind of "forgetting" similar to hysterical evasion. Behind all this we see primitive flight from danger, or the automatic avoidance called "primal repression" by Freud (1915, p. 148). Repression proper is considered a relatively late, post-oedipal form of defense (A. Freud, 1936). Similarly, even the most primitive forms of repression scored in the MCT are not typical of our youngest and most immature children, where even simpler avoidance strategies prevail.

We have discussed the development of defense as if one stage necessarily follows the other. As a matter of fact, we know little about how far these developments can be "bent" by variations in the home environment, or by therapy. The kind of data accumulated in our study gives us little basis for such speculations. Although the youngest subjects were similar in their use of primitive defensive strategies, they clearly differed with respect to their preferred strategies, with one child choosing flight, another denial, and another primitive isolation. These preferences may serve as starting points for diverging (or sometimes converging) chains of development. As far as more general trends of development are concerned, however, we believe the stage sequence presented here to be fairly representative, even if the relatively high percentage of children from academic families may have moved the points of transition downward.

It may be instructive to compare our developmental sequence with results obtained from a spiral aftereffect (SAE) test given to children aged 3;9 to 6;11 years (Andersson, Johansson, Karlsson, and Ohlsson, 1972). The youngest and cognitively most immature children registered very brief SAEs. According to Andersson et al., these children depended on extraceptive factors in their perceptions, thus blocking their production of the subjective SAE. The next stage was characterized by very long SAEs, implying a dependence on intraceptive (subjective) factors instead of extraceptive ones. In the most mature stage the intermediate SAE duration indicated decentering or a balance between inner and outer determinants. It is also interesting to note that children in the first stage did not comprehend the meaning of dreams, i.e., of a subjective world as opposed to an objective one. The parallels between these three stages and those described by us are striking (e.g., the inability of our youngest children to produce AIs, the preponderance of subjective projections in the middle groups, and the beginning self-nonself balance reached in the most mature children). The data collected by Andersson et al. in this and later studies (Andersson and Weikert, 1974) support the conclusion that our data reflect a fundamental developmental pattern. This pattern is congruent with the cognitive changes mapped by Piaget and others, but it also encompasses emotional aspects of growth.

MCT and AI protocols in older children and adults are usually scored with an eye to the position of a sign, early or late, in the series. A late sign is more likely to be linked to the present situation than a sign appearing only in early sections. Support for this assumption has been presented on several occasions (e.g., Smith, Sjöholm, and Nielzén, 1976). In our second study we did not differentiate between early and late signs, mainly because we were often unable to ascertain a stable C-phase in our subjects. A clear differentiation of the P-phase and C-phase levels is based on the elimination (and disqualification) of content (and modes of handling content) related to early levels. Many normal schoolchildren in fact did not eliminate all previous content (in the MCT) when new content emerged; instead they retained the old content together with the new material. In other words, in their constructions of outside reality they did try to keep the connections with previous stages as open as possible. One reason why signs of retention were not found in the preschool children could be, quite simply, that they consider retention too self-evident to report. But let us offer another explanation: retention may be a useful instrument for P-phase to C-phase transmission only when such a connection is being severed by the progressive separation of the two levels. In normal young children who lack a definite or stable C-phase, even early P-phases are likely to remain open to communication. To use more precise PG terminology, where reconstruction of P-phase content is not hampered by a well-defined C-phase level, retention is unnecessary.

Many childish response categories in the MCT have also been identified in older children and in adults — but as clearly psychotic manifestations. We particularly wish to mention drastic projections (of animals and extra people in the B-percept) and zero-phases. It seems almost self-evident that the more established the C-phase, the more disrupting a projective invasion or a breakdown of the percept is. Since drastic projections were mostly scored in the egocentric middle groups, one might speculate on whether adult paranoia implies a regression to this period, roughly corresponding to the oedipal period, when important social relations are established. The regressions reflected in schizophrenic zero-phases reach much further back, to stages where a well-defined reality contact is completely lacking. These and similar problems will be treated more thoroughly once the study of clinical children is presented.

PART TWO

COMPARISON WITH CLINICAL CHILDREN

4

PRESENTATION OF CLINICAL GROUP

The entire clinical group consisted of 75 subjects (45 boys and 30 girls) between 4 and 16 years of age.[1] In the original selection of patients from a child psychiatric clinic we avoided those who were older than 16 years but tried to include children as young as possible. No child suspected of organic lesion was accepted. Our subjects were primarily selected with an eye to symptoms of anxiety, although not necessarily severe symptoms. The subjects were free from medication during the testing period, except for a few cases where such treatment was absolutely necessary.

CLINICAL DESCRIPTION

As is well known to students of clinical psychology, diagnoses are unreliable criteria, frequently varying from one clinician to another. Therefore, the clinic staff was not asked for final diagnoses of the children but rather for as many concrete observations and impressions as possible. This caution with regard to the use of diagnostic classes, however, need not force us to abandon diagnostic concepts in considering the factorial groupings (Chapter 9).

There were originally 48 symptom dimensions, pertaining to near-psychotic or psychotic reactions, paroxysmal anxiety, phobic fears, school and separation anxiety, other specified fears, somatic symptoms, anticipations of disaster, self-destructive ten-

[1] The reader will remember that the normal group, used for comparison, included 127 subjects (60 boys and 67 girls) between 4 and 15 years of age.

99

dencies, typical individual reactions in frightening situations, passivity, hyperactivity, cognitive disturbances, regressive behavior, depressive manifestations, compulsive rituals, etc. All these dimensions are listed in Chapter 9.

Age Differences

Some of the important symptom dimensions are unevenly distributed over the different age levels. There were more near-psychotic subjects around puberty and more depressed ones among the younger children. This problem, together with other sampling problems, will be discussed in detail in Chapter 9. It may be argued that even if our anxiety-ridden children represent a good sampling of the nonorganic cases at a particular clinic, these cases do not necessarily reflect the general distribution of mental disturbances in the age groups under consideration. Yet it would be very surprising if the age differences with regard to some of the key symptoms were not mainly caused by true developmental differences.

METHOD

If it was considered advisable, the experimenter spent some time with the child at the clinic before the testing session. As a result, few children refused to be tested. In addition to the landscape test, we also used the AI test and the MCT as described before.

The test protocols were scored independently of the description of clinical symptoms, often long before any clinical data were available. In the presentation of the MCT in Chapter 1 the high interrater reliability was mentioned. The disagreements between the two raters were somewhat less for the clinical children than for the normal children. In the few cases of slight disagreement, the rater who had had no personal contact with the children or their therapists decided the final score. The AI scoring presented no problems.

All the 75 children will be used only in discussing the AI data (Chapter 5). In other chapters, as well as some tables in Chapter 5, the number of subjects will be slightly reduced. An obvious reason for this reduction is that subjects with truncated AI series or with insufficient clinical data have been excluded. Another reason is that at times we focus on the schoolchildren, narrowing the age span to 7–16 years.

LANDSCAPE TEST

Using the landscape test of cognitive egocentrism (Piaget and Inhelder, 1941, 1948), the children in each age group were characterized as either mature or immature (see Table 4.1). The younger the children were, the more decisive the cognitive task was for their placement in these subgroups (for details see Chapters 2 and 3). As in our initial study of schoolchildren, the 11-year-olds were divided into three groups, the most mature ones (with no landscape errors) being included in the group of 12- to 13-year-olds. Preschool children (under age 7) were divided into six subgroups, following the guidelines described in Chapter 3. Thus, to review briefly, group 1 consisted of children under 6 years with either no comprehension of the task at all (1a) or an incorrect answer even with regard to their own perspective (1b). Group 2 included children 5 to 6 years old, most of whom comprehended the task but still made one or more errors. Finally, group 3 included the older preschoolers, with subgroup 3a consisting of the children 5 years or older with all correct choices.

TABLE 4.1
DISTRIBUTION OF CLINICAL SUBJECTS

Age and cognitive maturity level	N
< 7 years old*	11
7–10(11) immature	12
7–10(11) mature	15
12–13 immature	3
(11)12–13 mature	13
14–16 immature	4
14–16 mature	17

* The various subgroups are not shown here as these did not prove to be particularly meaningful for the clinical preschool children.

In general, there were no great differences between the clinical and normal groups with respect to cognitive maturity (see Chapter 7).

AFTERIMAGE TEST

The AI test procedure has been described in Chapter 1. Details of the scoring dimensions will be presented in Chapter 5.

META-CONTRAST TECHNIQUE

The use of the MCT followed the guidelines established in Chapter 1. Many of the scoring dimensions have already been discussed in our presentation of the normal children (Chapters 2 and 3). Of particular relevance to the clinical group is a discussion of depressive tendencies (Chapter 6), signs of inadequate defenses (Chapter 7), and anxiety manifestations (Chapter 8).

5

AFTERIMAGE DATA

In our previous studies, we have used AIs to represent adaptive processes in normal and pathologically disturbed adults (Smith and Kragh, 1967; Andersson, Nilsson, Ruuth, and Smith, 1972). Chapters 2 and 3 presented our work with normal children 4 to 15 years of age. This chapter will trace signs of anxiety in the AI serials of the clinical children. We shall also closely scrutinize allied signs of primitive functioning and psychotic discontinuity. In Chapter 8 we will report on how the presence of depression in the clinical children implies that AI size diminishes from trial to trial.

SUBJECTS

An overview of the subjects can be gained from Table 5.1 (p. 107). The preschool children do not really concern us here since few of them could produce acceptable AI serials.

Certain differences in cognitive maturity should be mentioned here. In the two oldest groups shown in the table, some clinical subjects were unable to give completely correct answers on the landscape test. These subjects, who have no counterpart in the normal group, will be treated separately in most comparisons below. In the clinical group of younger schoolchildren, 12 were immature and 15 mature compared with 19 and 17, respectively, in the normal group. This slight intergroup difference will tend to work against our hypotheses.

SCORING DIMENSIONS

The relevant scoring dimensions for the AI test will be described in relation to the various research problems discussed below. At this point, however, it seems helpful to present the dimensions used in comparisons with clinical symptoms and MCT results.

CLINICAL SYMPTOMS

As noted in Chapter 4, the clinical children were rated on the presence or absence of a number of symptoms. In our classification of anxiety dimensions we have relied on Anthony (1975c), among others. The following dimensions will concern us here:

1. *Paroxysmal anxiety:* Acute attacks of anxiety, panic, other sudden and uncontrollable outbreaks, feelings of approaching disaster.

2. *Chronic anxiety:* A chronic state of high tension, several somatic symptoms or particularly severe symptoms such as persistent food refusal or vomiting, anticipation of something unpleasant or other apprehensions and "worries."

3. *Focused anxiety:* Unnecessary fright of particular persons or situations (including both phobias and pseudo-phobias).

4. *More diffuse anxiety reactions:* Minor somatic symptoms such as sleep disturbances, enuresis, nail biting, scratching, or stomach upsets.

We also noted signs of *cognitive disturbances* in the subject's *contact with reality.* (Since clear signs of paroxysmal anxiety and of disturbed contact with reality were comparatively rare in the clinical group, we also accepted slightly uncertain signs as indicative of the presence of these disturbances.)

META-CONTRAST TECHNIQUE

The reader is asked to accept the validity of the following scoring dimensions pending more detailed analysis in later chapters:

1. *Conventional signs of severe anxiety:* (a) The threat (A_2) and the hero (in B_2) are seen close together or are *fused;* (b) the defensive mechanisms are *"leaking"* (e.g., an "isolating" subject may see a curtain covering the area in B_2 where A_2 is being projected but, at the same time, sense something dangerous behind the curtain); (c) at least two *zero-phases* occur (i.e., reports where nothing or only

chaos is perceived by the subject); (d) *open fright* is expressed in the test situation; (e) *broken structures* (e.g., a picture falling to pieces) are reported.

2. *Openly expressed anxiety or feelings of impending disaster:* Signs of types (d) and (e) above represent this dimension. Because of the relative scarcity of these signs, we also accepted somewhat marginal signs.

3. *Discontinuity:* (a) Drastic projections are seen (i.e., the change in B [influenced by the subliminal A] is so great that it jeopardizes or actually breaks the continuity between the present report and the preceding one); (b) at least two zero-phases occur; (c) B is generally unstable or reported as different, although the difference is never defined (this sign was accepted only in combination with at least one zero-phase).

4. *Eye-shutting or avoidance behavior:* The subject shuts his own eyes or turns his head away when presented with the stimuli (a direct defensive reaction typical of the normal preschool children, except subgroup 3b).

PRIMITIVE FUNCTIONING

On the basis of our pilot studies, it could be predicted that the AIs of clinical children would show more primitive signs than those of normal children. Since we matched the comparison groups on performance on the landscape test, such a result could not be explained on the basis of the subjects' cognitive skills. The relative immaturity shown by the clinical children on the AI test should rather be viewed, from a broad functional-emotional perspective, as indicating the lack of articulation of their sense of self in relation to outside reality. In other words, the AI serials of these anxiety-ridden children were expected to show that they do not function at levels of self-articulation congruent with their age and actual cognitive ability, but prefer to regress to the relative ease and safety of more infantile levels, especially when confronted with a new adaptive task.

SCORING

In previous AI studies, primitive characteristics have been scored along dimensions of size, brightness, and color. Since many of our clinical subjects could make only crude estimates on the brightness scale, with emphasis on the dark end more than the light, "positive" one, we limited our scoring to size and color. (Reports of very bright, achromatic shades have always been scarce anyhow.) AIs were considered primitive if they were reasonably constant in size (≤ 6.5 cm) and/or positively colored (red, brown, yellow, reddish violet). We noted the presence of at least two small or two positive AIs in a serial. A few subjects saw nothing but primitive AIs, but the sample was too small for statistical comparisons. Instead, we have listed subjects who did not report any negative, chromatic (blue, blue-green) AIs.

RESULTS

Many significant differences between clinical and normal subjects appear in Table 5.1. Normal preschool children from subgroups 2a–3b were fairly successful in producing AIs whereas the corresponding clinical children were not. In schoolchildren the differences in the proportion of subjects with small AIs were particularly significant. Adding all subgroups (except cognitively immature subjects aged 12 or over), we find 29 clinical subjects with at least two small AIs and 20 without. The corresponding figures in the normal group are 12 and 57 ($\chi^2 = 22.23$, $df = 1$, $p < 0.001$, two-tailed, with calculations of exact probabilities for each age group also yielding significant values). We also find 26 clinical subjects and 11 normal subjects completely lacking negative, chromatic images ($\chi^2 = 19.89$; exact p values for the two oldest age groups were separately significant). It may be added that the most common size deviations in the 49 clinical subjects being compared here were in the direction of small AIs rather than large (≥ 11.0 cm) ones: 16 subjects were scored for small AIs only, 13 for small as well as large ones, three for large AIs alone.

COMMENTS

The first question to ask in relation to Table 5.1 is why the color difference between the groups did not involve the presence

TABLE 5.1

TRUNCATED, SIZE-CONSTANT, AND DIFFERENTLY COLORED AI SERIALS IN CLINICAL AND NORMAL CHILDREN*

Age and cognitive maturity level	Number of AI phases			≥2 AIs ≤6.5 cm		≥2 positive AIs		No negative, chromatic AIs		≥1 green AI	
	None	<8*	≥8	Yes	No	Yes	No	Yes	No	Yes	No
4–6											
1a + 1b	3 (14)	0 (2)	0 (4)	0 (4)	0 (0)	0 (2)	0 (2)	0 (4)	0 (0)	0 (0)	0 (4)
2a + 2b + 3a	4 (1)	2 (5)	1 (21)	0 (19)	1 (4)	1 (8)	0 (15)	0 (14)	1 (8)	0 (1)	1 (22)
3b	0 (1)	0 (0)	1 (6)	0 (6)	1 (0)	0 (2)	1 (4)	0 (4)	1 (2)	0 (0)	1 (6)
7–10(11) immature	3 (2)	1 (0)	8 (17)	8 (7)	0 (10)	3 (6)	5 (11)	3 (4)	5 (13)	1 (5)	7 (12)
7–10(11) mature	0 (0)	2 (1)	13 (16)	7 (3)	6 (14)	2 (9)	11 (7)	7 (4)	6 (12)	2 (5)	11 (11)
12–13 immature***	0	0	3	3	0	3	0	2	1	1	2
(11)12–13 mature	1 (0)	1 (1)	11 (16)	6 (1)	5 (15)	1 (6)	10 (10)	6 (0)	5 (16)	1 (10)	10 (7)
14–16 immature	0	0	4	2	2	0	4	2	2	2	2
14–16 mature	0 (0)	0 (0)	17 (19)	8 (1)	9 (18)	4 (6)	13 (13)	10 (3)	7 (16)	1 (5)	16 (14)

* Figures within parentheses represent the normal group.

** As in Table 3.2, incomplete serials were used in the other columns only if the data permitted a definite conclusion about the serial had it been complete.

*** There is no comparison group in the normal children.

of positive colors as much as an absence of negative hues. In a typical normal AI protocol with positive AIs, one usually also finds negative AIs. In a clinical protocol, one finds, instead, a mixture of positive and achromatic hues or only the latter. If we consider achromatic shades as a compromise between positive and negative tendencies, we may well label achromatic AI serials as immature. It also seems likely that in children with manifest anxiety the darkness of the AI tends to render color discrimination particularly difficult and tempts them to report only the darkness (see below).

The higher frequency of truncated AI serials in the clinical group is not a new finding. Relating it to previous findings in adult subjects (Smith and Sjöholm, 1974b), we may consider it a sign of anxiety—the only such sign supplied by the AI test for our young and cognitively immature clinical subjects. Children with symptoms of anxiety are generally more agitated and less patient, have greater difficulties in fixating the projection screen, are more often frightened of the AI phenomenon itself, and are more uncertain about how to define the AI in relation to themselves and physical reality—all circumstances rendering it difficult for the child to hold the AI for inspection.

ANXIETY

In our initial study of normal schoolchildren (Chapter 2), we used a number of anxiety signs (adapted from work with adults) and pertaining to the size and the darkness of the AI. In that study, however, we decided not to score large AIs as anxiety signs when they appeared in serials which probably reflected a generally unstable self-nonself relation rather than manifest anxiety; we thus did not score large AIs in serials that also included size-constant AIs. In contrast, with the clinical group, because of the sizable number of serials with one or more small AIs, we had to consider large AIs in all serials.

Our earlier use of primitive AIs as a sign of anxiety in more mature children was suggested by a factor-analytic study of adults (Smith, Fries, Andersson, and Ried, 1971), in which the anxiety factor was found to be highly loaded with primitive signs. As stated before, truncated serials are also likely to reflect anxiety. Among the severe anxiety signs listed above for the MCT are zero-phases, particularly in children (11)12 years or older. Analogous signs in the AI test would be so-called real regressions to small or more physiognomic AIs (for a detailed description, see the next section). We omitted color regressions (because some color reports in the normal group proved too ambiguous to be used here) and brightness regressions (because many clinical subjects could not use the brightness scale).

SCORING

1. *Established anxiety signs:* (a) At least three AIs ≥ 10.5 cm in serials without size-constant (≤ 6.5 cm) AIs; (b) at least two AIs estimated as ≥ 10 on the brightness scale or described as dark or black; or, instead of one such AI, two achromatic AIs estimated as 9, three chromatic AIs estimated as 10, or two large AIs.

2. *Primitive signs:* At least five positive AIs and/or size-constant AIs in subjects at the two upper age and cognitive maturity levels.

3. *Regressions:* At least one real regression (see next section) from a mature AI level to an immature one in subjects at the two upper age and cognitive maturity levels (again, color and brightness regressions were not considered).

4. *New anxiety signs:* Signs of type (1a) above in serials with size-constant AIs.

5. *Truncated serials:* At least three phases totally lacking.

RESULTS AND COMMENTS

The immature clinical subjects aged 12 and above have been omitted from Table 5.2, as have the preschool children (the only characteristic of most clinical preschool children is their inability to produce AIs). Not considering the incomplete AI serials in column 5, we find 38 clinical subjects with anxiety signs and 11 without, compared with 30 and 38 normal subjects, respectively ($\chi^2 = 13.08$, $df = 1$, $p < 0.001$, two-tailed). With the incomplete serials included the χ^2 value increases to 15.16. Scoring category 3 (regressions) plays a subordinate role here.

Understandably, the difference between the normal and clinical groups seems to be least marked during puberty.

TABLE 5.2
AI SIGNS OF ANXIETY IN CLINICAL AND NORMAL CHILDREN*

Group	1 Established anxiety signs	2 Rest with primitive signs	3 Rest with regressions	4 Rest with new signs	Σ1-4	5 Truncated serials	6 Complete serials — no anxiety
7–10(11) immature	2 (6)	—	—	4 (2)	6 (8)	4 (2)	2 (9)
7–10(11) mature	10 (5)	—	—	3 (0)	13 (5)	2 (1)	0 (11)
(11)12–13 mature	3 (4)	5 (3)	0 (0)	0 (0)	8 (7)	2 (1)	3 (9)
14–16 mature	6 (5)	4 (4)	1 (0)	0 (1)	11 (10)	0 (0)	6 (9)

* Figures in parentheses represent the normal group.

Regarding the more pronounced difference at the age level just below ([11]12–13 years), we would like to refer back to Table 5.1, where 10 of the 17 subjects in the normal group were scored for green color but only one in the clinical group of 11 received this score ($p = 0.02$, Fisher's exact test, two-tailed). As has been mentioned several times, clearly green color reported in the AI experiment is likely to be a sign of isolation as a defensive strategy. This is compatible with the description of the normal prepubescent child as "a mildly obsessive child whose compulsions are very likely to pass with the onset of puberty" (Anthony, 1975b, p. 372). Children with manifest anxiety obviously lack the benefit of this normal defense.

In order to inquire more closely into the power of the signs in Table 5.2, we divided the clinical subjects according to the types of observed anxiety symptoms: paroxysmal or chronic anxiety, on the one hand, and less severe anxiety, on the other. The special signs used to characterize AIs at the upper age levels have been recorded separately, and the primitive signs have been strengthened by including only completely primitive serials (Table 5.3). In view of the severity of the corresponding MCT signs (zero-phases), we have also judged real AI regressions to be particularly severe signs. Unfortunately, the sample of younger schoolchildren was smaller than one might have wished and they are rather unevenly divided by the anxiety symptom scale. In the older age groups, we find that the number or severity of anxiety signs correlates with the clinical severity of anxiety. Signs of primitive functioning seem to play a more prominent role in this correlation than do signs of regression. The difference between subjects with severe anxiety and all other subjects emerges very clearly ($\chi^2 = 25.83$, $df = 2$, $p < 0.0005$, one-tailed).

Psychotic Discontinuity

Signs of regression played a rather marginal role in differentiating between normal and clinical subjects and between subjects with more or less severe anxiety symptoms. One reason was that subjects with regressions often showed other anxiety signs as well (Table 5.2); another was that color regressions had

TABLE 5.3

AI SIGNS OF ANXIETY AND SEVERITY OF ANXIETY SYMPTOMS

Anxiety signs in AI test	7–10(11) immature			7–10(11) mature			12–16 immature			(11)12–16 mature		
	Severe anxiety	Mild anxiety	Normal group	Severe anxiety	Mild anxiety	Normal group	Severe anxiety	Mild anxiety	Normal group	Severe anxiety	Mild anxiety	Normal group
Truncated serials	1	2	2	2	0	0	0	0	–	1	0	0
Dark/large AIs	1	5	8	9	3	5	1	2	–	11	2	10
Only size-constant	–	–	–	–	–	–	–	–	–	3	0	0
Only positive ± achromatic	–	/	–	–	–	–	–	–	–	5	0	0
Real regressions	–	–	–	–	–	–	–	–	–	5	0	0
≥2 signs or regressions	–	–	–	–	–	–	–	–	–	10	0	0
1 sign, no regressions	1	4	8	9	3	5	1	2	–	7	2	10
No signs	0	2	7	0	2	2	1	6	–	3	6	26

to be excluded for the technical reasons noted above. Nevertheless, we decided to look more closely into the significance of signs of regression, not only as indicators of manifest anxiety but, like the zero-phases in the MCT, as markers of psychotic discontinuity. It has already been demonstrated that AI serials in adult schizophrenics are characterized by regressions and that the probability of regression increases with the severity of the psychopathology (Smith, Ruuth, Franzén, and Sjöholm, 1972). We also wished to clarify the diagnostic difference between protocols characterized by intermittent regressions to primitive AIs and protocols with nothing but primitive AIs.

In view of the greater likelihood of partial primitive functioning in young and cognitively immature subjects, even normal ones, we decided to limit our analysis to the two older age groups (excluding the immature 12- to 13-year-olds). Because of the small number of subjects with regressions, we decided to accept one (or more) real regression as indicative of severe discontinuity and two (or more) pseudo-regressions as indicative of more marginal cases (eventually these were included in a single regression group). The difference between the two kinds of regression will be made clear below.

SCORING

1a. *Real regression:* Change occurs from a mature AI to an immature one, i.e., from size ≥ 8.0 cm to size ≤ 6.5 cm; from negative to positive color; from an AI reflecting the meaning of the stimulus (the AI was most often reported as a mere oval, sometimes as a schematic face) to an AI reflecting another, more concrete or physiognomic meaning ("a giraffe," "a laughing face," "a Christmas tree"). For obvious reasons, the brightness dimension could not be used for scoring regression. Real regressions should occur from one phase to the next in serials where the initial phase is not primitive.

1b. *Pseudo-regression:* The first phase is primitive in the same way as the regression phase; or one or two phases intervene between the normal phase and the regression phase; or the regression occurs "within" one and the same phase.

2. *Completely primitive serials:* All phases are constant in size or positive.

3. *The rest:* The remainder of the sample without these signs.

RESULTS

To understand the details of Table 5.4, the reader should refer to the MCT scoring categories presented at the beginning of this chapter. The intergroup differences can be summarized in the following way. Group 1 (real and pseudo-regression) differs from group 3 (the rest) with respect to symptoms of paroxysmal anxiety ($p = 0.001$, Fisher's exact test, one-tailed) and disturbed reality contact ($p = 0.004$). The primitive group remains somewhere below the median. Group 3 differs from the other two groups with respect to chronic anxiety ($p = 6 \times 10^{-5}$). Severe anxiety signs in the MCT are most common in the regression group and least common in group 3. The difference is more pronounced for MCT signs of open anxiety ($p = 10^{-4}$), the primitive group again drawing closer to group 3. A similar trend is true for discontinuity in the MCT, whereas eye-shutting behavior tends to be slightly less common in the real regression group (1a) than in the other three groups (the primitive group in particular).

COMMENTS

The groups thus distinguished by their AI serials have been defined by the clinical symptoms and the MCT signs in the following way. The *regression group* (both real and pseudo-regression) is characterized by paroxysmal anxiety as well as by many anxiety signs in the MCT, including signs of openly expressed anxiety. The presence of discontinuity in the MCT supports the picture of a severely dysfunctional group, clinically often suspected of disturbed reality contact. This group is in part resembled by the *primitive group,* but there are fewer signs of paroxysmal or openly expressed anxiety and the disturbed reality contact does not seem to bear so many near-psychotic characteristics. Another difference, unfortunately not statistically significant in our small sample, is the presence of infantile defensive strategies in this group (as shown in the MCT), strategies the subjects may fall back on when more sophisticated ones fail them.

TABLE 5.4
CLINICAL SYMPTOMS AND MCT DATA FOR THREE AI GROUPS AMONG
OLDER CLINICAL SUBJECTS

AI groups for subjects (11)12–13 mature and 14–16	Clinical Variables										MCT Variables					
	Paroxysmal anxiety		Chronic anxiety		Disturbed reality contact		Severe anxiety signs			Openly expressed anxiety		Discontinuity		Eye-shutting behavior	
	+	–	+	–	+	–	≥3 +	2 +	<2 +	+	–	+	–	+	–
1a (≥1 real regression)	4	1	5	0	4	1	2	1	2	4	1	4	1	1	4
1b (≥2 pseudo-regressions)	2	1	3	0	2	1	2	1	0	3	0	1	2	2	1
Σ1	6	2	8	0	6	2	4	2	2	7	1	5	3	3	5
2 (primitive)	2	6	8	0	5	3	0	4	4	2	6	2	6	6	2
3 (the rest)	1	16	6	11	2	15	0	2	15	1	16	2	15	7	10

* Figures to the left in a column represent the presence of a sign as defined in the test; figures to the right, its absence.

DISCUSSION

The existence of significant, often highly significant differences between the clinical and the normal children and between various subgroups within the clinical group proves that certain AI test phenomena are not spurious or unreliable. The differences seem all the more remarkable given the transitory character of most AIs and the difficulty in keeping children, particularly young and mentally disturbed ones, involved in a long and rather tedious task. The test's usefulness did not, however, extend to the preschool level in the clinical group. With normal children, the technique proved to be useful down to age 4 or 5 (Chapter 3).

Judging by previous reactions to our publications, many experimental psychologists regard our use of AIs as highly irregular. Such critics may claim that our results do not really pertain to AIs as perceptual phenomena but rather to the subject's idiosyncratic style of reporting or other artifacts of the specific experimental situation. Those who deny that AIs can have anything to do with processes beyond the perceiver's retina obviously have a very particular type of AI in mind—the AIs produced by adults and relatively mature children after sufficient practice in front of a projection screen. From our perspective, however, these AIs are secondary phenomena, rather useless for the study of personality. The more subjective adaptive process leading up to this isolated end-product has been largely ignored in classical experiments, or merely noted as expectable deviation.

Our own account of personality research based on the AI test does not make any claim to completeness. In Chapter 1, we mentioned the use of progressively diminishing AI size to characterize depressive retardation (see Chapter 6 for a detailed discussion). Another AI quality, color variegation, has been regarded as an indication of hypersensitivity or mild projective tendencies (Smith, Sjöholm, and Nielzén, 1974). Here variegation does not allude to the schematic features of the stimulus ("red eyes in a bluish oval"); it is free from narrow stimulus dependence ("the upper half red, the bottom part green," etc). In previous work the latter kind of report was found to correlate not only with clinical symptoms of hypersensitivity but also with signs of hypersensitivity in the MCT (changes in B while A is still subliminal). A similar correlation has been found in the present material (cf. Chapters 2 and 9, in particular).

The diagnostic dimensions treated in this chapter are all related to anxiety. Primitive AI signs seem to be typical of our anxiety-ridden children, not because they are cognitively retarded but because they choose to function at levels lagging behind their cognitive development. Their preference for a less advanced and therefore less demanding level of functioning is apparently one side of their general strategy to avoid, or at least reduce the impact of, anxiety-provoking situations. The more articulated and complex the adaptive demands on a person, the greater the risk is that anxiety signals will be recognized, that the possibility of danger will penetrate into consciousness. As we shall see below, defensive regression does not follow the same pattern in all individuals; it may also be more or less successful as an anxiety-reducing strategy.

First, however, let us summarize the AI signs of manifest anxiety. Like adults, children and adolescents reveal their anxiety in enlarged and darkened images. As we go down the age and cognitive maturity scale, we find that dark and black AIs become more prominent as an expression of anxiety at the perceptual level. One apparent reason is the inveterate tendency of immature AIs to remain size-constant. In the older children AI regressions were also considered indirect, but reliable, signs of anxiety. Another anxiety indicator was young children's tendency to strangle their AI production altogether. We have encountered similar avoidance reactions in adults, particularly adults inclined to entertain all-or-nothing types of defense (Smith and Sjöholm, 1974b). With the clinical children, we prefer to associate such a reaction with infantile denial and perhaps suggest a developmental link between denial and compulsive defenses (cf. Chapter 7).

In considering defensive strategies, primitive defenses like denial, and apparently also regression, can be looked at as simultaneous indications of imminent anxiety because of the transitory, nonstructural character of the defense. The anxiety is not encapsulated forever by the defense, only momentarily avoided. In the case of depressive retardation, the initiating anxiety may be seen in the oversized AIs which dominate early phases of the adaptive process. With each new adaptive encounter, the anxiety is quenched once again by the retardation. In relation to the mild obsessions in prepuberty mentioned in connection with green images, anxiety seems to have disappeared altogether, perhaps to enable effective adaptation to outside realities before the onset of puberty (see Chapter 2). The presence of green color, then, is not here a sign of anxiety. Instead, the absence of this defense in the corresponding clinical group may probably be taken as a *mene tekel.*

As indicated in Table 5.4, there was a correlation between discontinuities in the AI process and symptoms of paroxysmal and openly expressed anxiety. Regressions both to immature AIs and to what Schur (1958) and Cameron (1963) have called primary anxiety were found in the same individuals. Knowing that paroxysmal anxiety, as opposed to neurotic signal anxiety, is likely to be a serious symptom (in subjects as old as ours), we shall try to better define the regression group by comparing it with the primitive group. Both groups were no doubt severely disturbed in many ways—but differently. The primitive subjects had regressed to a rather constant primitive level. They were also slightly more inclined to use infantile defenses in the MCT. The regression group did not seem to have such an established alternative. The regressions were intermittent and temporary; they seemed more like foreign intrusions in a still partly adequate functional pattern. Compared with their infantilized counterparts, these subjects showed more disintegrated (split) reactions; some of them were well on their way to schizophrenic development.

An interesting observation from the MCT protocols of three children in the regression group was their very early recognition of the threat, almost at the first paired presentation, followed very quickly by a denial of the premature discovery. This extreme sensitivity, as if borne from a constant apprehension of danger, allows denial to function as a preventive measure rather than as a defense. Similar reactions have been observed in early or marginal, often nonregressive, cases of schizophrenia (Nyman, 1975). It is instructive, then, to learn that such extreme sensitivity is not exclusive to the regression group but has been traced in one or two cases among primitive subjects (but nowhere else). This may indicate a deeper resemblance between the two groups than was accounted for by the surface differences.

Experimental psychologists may wonder about the relation between deviant AI reactions and eidetic imagery. Our experiments did not favor the production of eidetic images, as they entailed long and repeated fixations of a rather simple stimulus. An eidetic image is most likely to appear after a brief, "wandering" observation of a varied and interesting picture. Several children in our groups may have been able to form such images given optimal opportunities. There is no good reason, however, to assume that the propensity for eidetic imagery should differ between the normal and the clinical groups and thereby influence the results—which in any case are fully comprehensible in terms of cognitive maturity, anxiety, and defense.

6

DEPRESSIVE TENDENCIES

Many problems connected with depression in childhood and adolescence still remain to be solved. While some clinicians claim to have observed depression in childhood, even in infancy, others deny such a possibility and place the emergence of true depression in the latency period or later. The roots of depression and its various manifestations are also debated. There does, however, appear to be growing agreement that depressive reactions in childhood and in adulthood, although distinct in many ways, form a developmental continuity (see Anthony, 1975a). Accepting this assumption in a very general way, we shall now try to throw light on some stages in the development of depression from the postoedipal period (5–6 years) until adolescence (14–16 years).

The AI test has previously been used to describe one of the core symptoms of adult depression — retardation (Smith, Kragh, Eberhard, and Johnson, 1970). It has also been known for some time (Smith and Kragh, 1967) that patients suffering from anxiety tend to produce oversized, often very dark, AIs. This finding was corroborated in the material reported in Chapter 5. In adult patients characterized by anxiety as well as depressive retardation, such oversized AIs were more likely to appear at the beginning of a series of AI productions than at the end. In other patients, characterized by anxiety and a depressive mood but not by retardation, AIs tended instead to become larger over trials. Thus, depressive retardation seemed to be specifically related to successive reduction of AI size.

These findings have been validated in two more recent studies (Smith, Fries, Andersson, and Ried, 1971; Smith, Sjöholm, and Nielzén, 1976). In these studies measurements of

121

AI size were combined with estimations of AI darkness. The larger and darker the AI, the more likely it was that it indicated anxiety. The retardation seen in the AI test obviously counteracted the black, threatening image that covered most of the projection screen by gradually making it smaller and, often at the same time, better delineated and lighter. Comparable results were obtained in the first of the above studies on a serial spiral aftereffect test (see also Andersson, Nilsson, Ruuth, and Smith, 1972).

Retardation in the AI series correlated not only with appropriate clinical criteria but also with signs of depressive stereotypy in the MCT (which should not be confused with primitive stereotypy as described in Chapter 2). Here, we wish to point out that the development toward correct recognition of A_2 within the frame of B_2 may be arrested by a series of stereotyped repetitions of incorrect reports (getting stuck like a broken record). Such stereotypies have been shown to reflect depressive states in the perceiver; the more marked or drawn-out the stereotypy, the more likely it is that it reflects depressive retardation.

In considering the problem of depression in our group of clinical children, two questions stand out: (1) Can our descriptive tools be applied to children at or before school age without considerable loss of power and precision? (2) If the answer is affirmative, how does depression manifest itself at different age levels in a sample of normal children and in clinical children generally characterized by anxiety? Our inclusion of the normal children indicates that we do not consider depressive reactions to be exclusively clinical problems. On the contrary, the strategies observed in depressive protocols may well be accentuated reflections of more common reactions to mental discomfort.

Since we have already found both the AI test and the MCT useful for diagnostic purposes in children, we would expect an affirmative answer to our first question. As far as the second question is concerned, we presumed that signs of depression and depressive retardation, although never deviating so far from adult signs as to be unrecognizable, would show at least some distinctively childish features consistent with the child's maturity level, i.e., the child's cognitive-emotional grasp of his own self in relation to outside reality. Examples of such changes in the development of various other defensive strategies have already been presented.

It is not, however, enough to state that we intend to follow depressive manifestations from a cognitive-developmental perspective. We are also looking at *processes*. What we are attempting is to see depression as a quality characterizing certain processes through which our subjects try to master their life situations. The process view has proved to be very fruitful for diagnostic-descriptive purposes. It should be noted, however, that the process view and the choice of instrumentation consistent with it imply that we put more emphasis on the formal side of depression, the retardation-inhibition complex, than is usually done in dynamic literature, and also on general problems of personality functioning.

Subjects

Of the 72 normal schoolchildren (7–15 years), 69 completed the AI test, and, of the 55 normal preschoolers (4–6 years), 31 did so. MCT data were secured for all 127 subjects. Of the 62 clinical schoolchildren (39 boys, 23 girls) who could be considered for this particular study, 31 boys and 22 girls completed the AI test. From the group of 10 clinical preschoolers (4 boys, 6 girls), only one (a boy) completed the test. All of these clinical subjects underwent the MCT and the landscape test.

The central symptom in all clinical subjects designated depressive was *a striking inability to experience joy and happiness;* in most cases this was associated with an extreme lack of self-confidence. Other symptoms recorded in varying degrees were signs of deep sadness, apathy, immobility, passivity, and the like. In addition to these core symptoms of depression, our children showed a number of more age-specific and indirect symptoms, such as aggression (in the more immature children), restlessness, and hyperactivity.

One group showed clear signs of depression. In other subjects, these signs were combined with manic components or with very obvious compulsive rituals. The reason the latter children were not included in the depressed group will be discussed below. Another group with marginal signs of depression was also evaluated separately, as were those few subjects for whom reliable clinical information regarding depression was unobtainable (referred to as "inadequate information" in Tables 6.2 and 6.3).

METHOD

SCORING RETARDATION IN THE AI TEST

As we have seen, the original method of determining retardation in an AI series was to find out whether a large image (≥ 11.0 cm) — which supposedly reflects anxiety — appeared among the early measurements, and was then followed by smaller images (Smith, Kragh, Eberhard, and Johnson, 1970). The method used in the cross-validation studies (Smith, Fries, Andersson, and Ried, 1971) included both measurements of size and estimations of darkness (1–10) for 15 consecutive trials. The dimensions of size and darkness were kept separate. Retardation could not be expected to always dominate the latter part of the serial in its entirety. Returns to high values had to be anticipated. With this in mind, we used consecutive values of linear regression (R) to describe retardation tendencies in the curves. These R-values covered the regression over five phases each; they overlapped in the following way: R_1 was based on phases 1–5, R_2 on phases 4–8, R_3 on phases 7–11, etc. All possible sequences of consecutive R-values were then tested until the sequence yielding the largest positive or negative sum had been found. Finally, the dominating sequence for size and the dominating sequence for darkness were considered together to find the main overall trend.

Since estimations of darkness were rather approximate in some of our subjects, we computed only size values. If more than two size measurements of the 10 in the standard series were missing in a child's protocol, his AI data were omitted from further consideration.

Using the least square method, the slope (M) of the series of size data was computed according to the equation

$$y = Mx + b$$

where $b = y$ intercept. Three possibilities were considered: (1) M is positive. In this case, no further computations were needed, and the series was labeled "nonretarded." (2) M is negative and at least -0.20, a value representing the approximate, lower quartile of all Ms in the present clinical sample. This value was not considered indicative of retardation in cases where the last five values of the AI series had a positive slope with a value (m) greater than M, i.e., where the general trend of the curve was strongly contradicted by the final trend. (3) M is negative, but not strongly so, i.e., less than 0.20. This value was disqualified by any positive value of m.

Other, more complicated computations, similar to those employed in previous studies, were also carried out. The conclusion was that the simple method just presented did not seem to misrepresent our empirical data.

Scoring Depression in the MCT

As we already pointed out, reports of negative AIs in adults correlate with so-called stereotypies in the MCT, i.e., reports in one trial after another of something (most often something not clearly understood) seen at the section of B_2 (the window) coinciding with the projected A_2. Stereotypies where one part of B_2 (most often the window) is perceived before the rest do not clearly correlate with depression, but are often found in adult primitive hysterics, who are inclined to resort to something close-at-hand in order to account for their impression of two-step exposures. Finally, in some adult depressives, A_2 is reported as *very* old, sick, or decrepit.

Using these results with adult subjects, we have tried to construct suitable scoring dimensions for our sample of children:

1. *Core signs:* (a) *Stereotypy,* or unchanged repetitions occurring at least five times in a row, with the subject reporting an incorrect A_2 within the frame of B_2. A_2 did not have to be vague ("something in the window," "a spot," etc.) but could have a definite meaning ("a

tree," "a house," "a young person," etc). In other words, we expected children's stereotypies to be less empty than those most often found in adults. (b) *Reports that the hero was injured* — a sign we felt obliged to connect with depression in our young subjects. (c) *Reports that A₂ was sick,* etc. (not encountered in our group).

2. *Marginal signs:* (a) *Primitive stereotypy,* or at least four unchanged repetitions or reports that the window in B_2 appears before the rest of B_2 on the screen (note the difference from ordinary stereotypies described above). (b) *Reports that A₂ was old* (a rather common sign among children). (c) *Reports that the hero was sad* (also a common sign).

RESULTS

In Table 6.1 negative AI trends are seen to be most closely associated with clear stereotypies in the MCT. A chi-square test, based on the italicized figures, yields a value of 7.36 ($df = 2$, $p < 0.025$, one-tailed); the exact p (using the fourfold contrast between the italicized upper left and the rest of the table) is 0.011 (one-tailed). The G-index of agreement reflecting the level of correlation expressed by that contrast reaches a value of $+ 0.41$. If, however, we compare the two left columns in the table, we notice that the covariation does not seem to increase with the magnitude of the negative M. The five exceptions at the lower left include the three most extreme M values ($- 0.50$ or below). Extreme negative Ms are likely to be found in AI series with late, sudden "regressions" to very small size values (a general sign of discontinuity rather than a particular sign of retardation). Aside from this, it should be mentioned that not only does a negative AI curve imply diminishing anxiety, operationally speaking, but also that few of the pronounced anxiety signs in the MCT (open fright in the test situation, defenses leaking anxiety, fusion of the threat and the hero) appear with stereotypy.

Table 6.1 will serve as the prototype for the choice of comparison groups in the following tables. One exception is the sign "hero injured," which we predicted would be a sign of depression but not particularly a sign of retardation (despite the fact that the only such sign entered in the table came from a child with a negative AI trend).

TABLE 6.1

MCT DEPRESSIVE SIGNS AND AI RETARDATION IN CLINICAL GROUP

MCT Signs	AI Trends					
	1 Negative M ≥ 0.20 (no positive $m > M$)	2 Negative M < 0.20 (no positive m)	Σ 1-2	3 Rest with a negative M or m	4 Rest without signs 1-3	Σ 3-4
Clear stereotypy	5	4	9(1)*	3	1	4(1)
Hero injured	0	1		0	0	
Hero sad	1	1		2	0	
A₂ old	1	2		2	2	
Primitive stereotypy	0	0	6(5)	4	0	10(7)
Rest without above signs	5	1	6(2)	11	8	19(6)

* Figures within parentheses refer to the number of subjects with severe anxiety signs in the MCT.

In Table 6.2, we find a significant agreement between a negative AI trend and clinical symptoms of depression without compulsive rituals or manic components. The exact p for this fourfold contrast yields a value of 6×10^{-5} (one-tailed) and the G-index of agreement is $+0.57$. If the italicized figures in the table are used, the corrected χ^2 is 21.25 ($df = 4$, $p < 5 \times 10^{-4}$, one-tailed). The size of the χ^2 indicates that the marginal or mixed forms of depression often correspond to AI series with mixed trends.

TABLE 6.2
AI RETARDATION AND CLINICAL SYMPTOMS OF DEPRESSION

Clinical Symptoms	AI Trends				
	1 Negative M ≥ 0.20 (no positive $m > 0.20$)	2 Negative M < 0.20 (no positive m)	Σ 1–2	3 Rest with negative M or m	4 Rest without signs 1–3
Depression (no rituals or manic components)	6	6	*12*	2	*0*
Depression (no rituals, etc.)	0	1		1	1
Depression + rituals	2	0		8	1
Depression with manic components	1	0		3	0
Σ marginal signs			*4*	*12*	*2*
No depression	1	2	*3*	*4*	*8*
Inadequate information	2	0		4	1

In Table 6.3 real stereotypy in the MCT correlates with clear depression. The exact p for the fourfold contrast is 3×10^{-4} and the G-index, $+0.53$. Calculation of a corrected χ^2 using the italicized figures produces a lesser value (11.61) than in Table 6.2, but it is still significant ($df = 4$, $p = 0.01$, one-tailed). Apparently, the weak or mixed symptoms correspond to the marginal, less marked signs in the MCT.

If we combine the AI and MCT tests (in 47 subjects, see Table 6.2), the test-symptom correlation is appreciably enhanced. With clear signs in at least one test and nonmarginal symp-

TABLE 6.3
MCT DEPRESSIVE SIGNS AND CLINICAL SYMPTOMS OF DEPRESSION

Clinical Symptoms	MCT Signs							
	1 Real stereotypy	2 Hero injured	Σ 1-2	3 Primitive stereotypy	4 Hero sad/A₂ old		Σ 3-4	5 Rest of sample
Depression (no rituals or manic components)	12	1	13	0	0	3	3	5
Depression (no rituals, etc.)	1	0		1	0	0		2
Depression + rituals	2	1		2	0	1		7
Depression with manic components	0	0		1	0	0		4
Σ marginal signs			4				5	13
No depression	2	1	3	1	3	4	8	10
Inadequate information	1	0		1	0	0		6

toms of depression defined as plus poles, the fourfold matrix yields a Fisher's exact p of 10^{-6} ($df = 1$, one-tailed) and a G-index of $+0.66$.

There seems to be a difference in the expected direction (although not a very pronounced one) between the proportions of negative AI trends in the normal and the clinical groups (strong trends appeared in 10% and 23%, respectively, of the school-age children [7 years or older]). The difference with respect to MCT stereotypy is clearly significant, with eight cases of stereotypy in the 72 normal schoolchildren and 18 cases in the 62 clinical schoolchildren ($\chi^2 = 6.84$, $df = 1$, $p < 0.005$, one-tailed).

It may also be worth noting that two maximums for negative AI trends appear in the normal group: one at age 5 to 6 and one at puberty (14–15). Of these subjects, 26% and 16%, respectively, had strong negative AI trends; only 8% of the other subjects showed such trends. In Chapters 2 and 3, it was shown that these two age groups, more than any others, were characterized by subjective inflation: the MCT reports of the young children were flooded with projected fantasies and the reports of the pubescent youngsters were colored by anxiety.

Even if we refrain from making quantitative comparisons *within* the clinical group, we consider it legitimate to discuss a few qualitative ones (in relation to the MCT). Table 6.4 indicates that uninterpreted stereotypy, hero duplication, "hero injured," and "A_2 old" are unevenly distributed over the different age-maturity groups.

DISCUSSION

As we noted earlier, there is still considerable disagreement among professionals regarding the existence of depression in childhood, as well as its symptomatology and etiology. However, most of those who doubt that depression is found in infancy and early childhood do appear to accept the presence of depressive signs in the postoedipal phase, i.e., the period with which our investigation here begins.[1]

---

[1] It might be noted that Abraham's (1911) "primal parathymia" refers to depressive feelings as early as the oedipal period.

TABLE 6.4
OVERVIEW OF MCT DEPRESSIVE SIGNS IN CLINICAL GROUP

MCT Hierarchy*	Age and Cognitive Maturity Groups					
	Preschool	7–10(11) immature	(11)12–13 immature	7–10(11) mature	(11)12–13 mature	14–16 all
Stereotypy: no definite meaning	0	0	1	0	1	3
Stereotypy: non-human object	0 (3)**	0 (2)	0	3 (1)	1	1
Stereotypy: adult human	0	0 (1)	0	0	0	1 (2)
Stereotypy: hero duplicate	0 (2)	4 (2)	1	2	0	0
Stereotypy: primitive	2 (2)	0	0	2	0	2
Hero injured	3	0	0	0	0	0
Hero sad	0 (1)	1	0	0	1	1
A_2 old	1 (1)	0	0	0	4	3
Rest of subjects without above signs	4 (46)	6 (14)	0	8 (16)	6 (17)	10 (17)

* Subjects scored and used up in the hierarchical order.
** Figures within parentheses refer to the normal subjects.

Sandler and Joffe (1965) have described a basic psychobiological reaction to mental pain rather early in childhood, although they emphasize that this reaction should not be confused with depressive illness. In our empirical study, however, such a differentiation did not seem decisive. Instead, we would agree with Mendelson (1974), who, after carefully reviewing the clinical literature, concluded that long-lasting states of depressive illness *do* occur in childhood and are overlooked or are diagnosed as something else. Mendelson's cases show some of the core symptoms listed by Lehmann (1959): sadness, drive reduction, retardation of expressive motor responses, etc. Yet one should keep in mind Sandler and Joffe's (1965) caution about using adult melancholia as a starting point for the investigation of childhood depression.

In discussing the probable etiology of depression, most dynamically oriented clinicians agree that early experiences of deprivation, neglect, or loss are key factors (Malmquist, 1972). Edward Bibring's (1953) emphasis on the loss of self-esteem, however, has been criticized by Mahler (1961), Rie (1966), and others as being inconsistent with the embryonic state of the child's self-concept. In this regard, we see "loss of psychological well-being" (Sandler and Joffe, 1965) as a more accurate description of narcissistic precursors of depression because it is more consistent with the undeveloped "representational world" of the young child.

Any consideration of etiology must also take into account the possibility of biological determinants. Engel and Schmale (1972), for example, have described a basic conservation-withdrawal regulatory process found in most animals. Their ideas serve as a tempting platform for speculations about a normal depressive reaction, of which depressive illness is but a pathological variant. Here, too, we find support for Sandler and Joffe's postulation of a basic psychobiological reaction (see also Schulterbrandt and Raskin, 1977).

Our own examination of depression may have been biased in at least two ways: (1) The depressive test signs were originally based on studies of adults, although we introduced variations of these signs to fit our young subjects. (2) Our clinical subjects were not primarily chosen with an eye to depressive states. The profile presented by our depressives is thus not very pronounced, although these subjects' symptom pictures very closely resemble the depressive reactions described by Sandler and Joffe (1965). Moreover, the clinical observations proved surprisingly reliable, judging from the intercorrelations.

At this point, we should explain why we did not include subjects with obsessive-compulsive rituals and manic symptoms in the main group of depressives. An earlier investigation using PG methods (Eberhard, Johnson, Nilsson, and Smith, 1965) showed beyond doubt that the presence of compulsive defenses blotted out a depressive profile in the test data. It would seem that obsessive isolation and control of affect render the particular "curbing" strategy in depression superfluous, at least in part. As Anthony (1975a) points out: "When depression is signaled, obsessive magical controls may be involved to compensate for feelings of helplessness, [and] hypomanic excitement to overcome lack of energy" (p. 265). Our cases with mixed symptoms did, however, show at least some correlation with the marginal signs in the AI test.

The correlations between the AI test and the MCT, on the one hand, and the clinical criteria, on the other, were quite high, considering all the uncontrollable variables expected to impair the reliability of our data (and, in the case of extremely negative AI curves, their validity). The difference between the normal and the clinical groups was most pronounced in the MCT. There was also a significant correlation between the two tests, especially between all instances of "real" stereotypy in the MCT and negative (but not extremely negative) trends in the AI series. Among the more marginal signs, "A is old" did not, as an isolated sign, correlate positively with clinical symptoms. In the previous studies of adult groups, comparable signs were generally more accentuated ("A$_2$ is sick," "decrepit," "dead," etc.).

Before discussing developmental trends in the picture of depression emerging from our test data, we need to analyze more closely the meaning of hero duplication in the MCT and the stereotypy associated with it. That is, we need to look at the tendency in some children to report in one trial after another, in a stereotyped way, that they perceive a playmate or another boy in the window (instead of the threatening A_2). Hero duplication can, first of all, be interpreted as an introjection of the threat or, more specifically, as a projected introjection (see Kragh, 1969; Andersson and Weikert, 1974). Since the introject closely resembles the hero, we see it as a narcissistic defense. In Chapter 2, we noted that hero duplication was particularly common at early school age. A combination of hero duplication and stereotypy would therefore be a more expectable occurrence at this age level than later. In line with this, stereotyped hero duplication was scored, above all, in the 7- to 10-year-olds.

To avoid dismissal of this combination as a statistical triviality, two points should be emphasized: (1) Stereotypy does not necessarily *combine* with hero duplication, even if the subject has been scored for that sign at some place in his percept genesis. In normal subjects, as pointed out in Chapter 2, reports of hero duplication are often repeated—but not in a stereotyped manner. (2) Most subjects with hero-duplication stereotypies employ other defensive strategies that might easily lend themselves to stereotyped repetition: reports of animals or objects, of nonthreatening persons (other than duplicates of the hero), of meaningless spots, etc. These kinds of stereotyped reports are often seen in other subjects.

We have already mentioned that many writers see a close relationship between depression and narcissistic injury. In her discussion of libido distribution, Anna Freud (1970) maintains that increased narcissism is the natural countermove to depressive neglect of the self. The stereotyped repetition of a narcissistically colored introject may be an attempt to bolster a "weakened" self, an attempt simultaneously marked by beginning depressive retardation. In Chapter 2, we speculated that primitive stereotypy might be a variant of the normal, unstereotyped tendency to repeat themes of hero duplication. This may explain why primitive stereotypy is a rather weak sign of depression.

Viewing our data from a developmental perspective, we now venture the following interpretations:

1. We have ample reason to believe, after many investigations, that a negative AI trend frequently represents a successive counteraction to tendencies to self-inflation. According

to our data, such a reaction is not uncommon among normal children and adolescents. Moreover, this finding occurs most often in periods of subjective expansion and anxiety (ages 5–6 and 14–15). This tempering tactic may be conceptualized as a basic response (Sandler and Joffe, 1965) and may serve both as an adaptive corrective and a defense against rising anxiety.

2. We cannot agree with those clinicians who consider childhood depression to be entirely different from adult depression. The core signs in both our tests correlate with clinical criteria over ages from about 7 to 16, at which point the MCT signs become more or less indistinguishable from adult signs (see below). Yet, although our data do seem to reflect basic structural similarities across a wide range, they also reflect important developmental differences in the experience of depression (see Anthony, 1975a), mostly qualitative differences.

The AI data in the normal group and results from both the AI test and the MCT in the clinical group indicate that signs of depression can be found at least as early as the postoedipal phase, and after age 7 these signs become very distinct. If depression is closely related to a narcissistic injury, we would expect our youngest children to visualize the threat to self in a very concrete way — as if the threat were physical. Although few young children were included in our analysis, it was only in this age group that the hero was reported to be injured (see Anna Freud, 1970). As defensive strategies become more internalized, concrete references to an injured body would be expected to disappear. In their place it seems the children (particularly, cognitively less mature children around 7 to 8 years of age) try to counter narcissistic blows by repeatedly projecting an image of themselves in the MCT. The stereotyped repetition of this apparently reveals the beginnings of depressive retardation. At the upper age levels in our clinical group, we did not find hero duplication. Stereotypies without any articulated content or meaning became more frequent. The picture of adult depression had emerged.

In summary, stereotypy in the MCT is for the most part limited to clinical cases of depression, where it obviously inhibits the most severe manifestations of anxiety. Taking into account the subjective side of these MCT responses, their content and meaning, we noted a close similarity between our subjects and adults only around early adolescence. Further down the age and cognitive maturity ladder, depression was more openly associated with countermeasures reflecting an underlying narcissistic injury. Adult depression seems an automatized, empty copy of the more direct childhood reaction.

Although negative regression in the AI test correlates with stereotypy in the MCT, as well as with clinical symptoms of depression, it seems to be a more general kind of response. It is typically found not only in adults but also in children below the age of 7. Nor is it exclusively confined to clinically depressed subjects; it is in fact generally scored in children at periods of subjective expansion (and danger from within). On the other hand, while the "depressive AI style" seems to reflect a moderately tempering influence in normal subjects, it correlates with a more obvious inhibition of mental functioning in the patient group. It would be tempting to conclude that the core reaction of depressive subjects—retardation—simply represents an exaggerated version of a relatively common defensive strategy.

7

INADEQUATE DEFENSES

The succession of defensive strategies in a PG series can be seen to present a developmental continuity. It was shown in Chapter 2 that strategies dominating late sections of the PG series of young children may also appear in the percept genesis of older children, but in the latter cases they are more likely to appear in much earlier sections (see Kragh, 1955). In other words, as percept genesis approaches the end-stage, primitive strategies are usually discarded in favor of more mature ones. The definition of defenses as more or less primitive here has generally been based on the age and cognitive maturity level at which they appear in normal development. If defensive strategies are defined in relation to either the subject's own percept genesis or data from different age-maturity strata, it will be possible to determine if a primitive strategy replaces a mature one in a later phase of the PG process. Such a shift will be termed regression.

As described in Chapter 2, extensive research has been done on the relation of defense mechanisms not only to age and cognitive maturity but also to specific personality configurations. In our previous work with adults, we encountered many MCT protocols where the effectiveness of various defenses seemed more than doubtful. Not until we started our systematic survey of defenses in children, however, did the ineffectiveness of some defensive structures become a crucial issue. In many children, most often those with symptoms of severe anxiety, these strategies could not fully mask, disguise, or bar the anxiety-tinged qualities of the perception, but allowed them to "leak through" the defensive fabric.

Let us say the subject reports a curtain in front of the window in B_2 where A_2 (the threat) is being projected. This is a common form of isolating defense. In this case, however, the subject glimpses something dark and frightening behind the curtain. Another subject may employ a repressive form of defense. Here A_2's threatening face is frozen into a lifeless mask, but big canine teeth come to fill the mouth of this decathected percept. In a third instance, the defects of the defensive system are not directly apparent in the perceptual report but are evident in the subject's behavior (e.g., a sudden gulping in of air). Another indication of anxiety at the behavioral level entails associations to something dangerous, repellent, or frightening.

In Chapter 2 such inadequate defenses were called *leaking mechanisms*. The study reported in that chapter suggested that leaking mechanisms are serious signs of a child's inability to come to terms with anxiety. Our emphasis here will not primarily be on the cross-validation of this tentative finding, but rather on how children with leaking defenses handle this situation, that is, which alternative means, if any, they choose to regain control. We thus plan to follow the child's percept genesis, starting with the phase in which the unreliability of the defense is first revealed and scrutinizing the subsequent phases for possible changes in the defensive strategy. If necessary, the PG process will be followed to its end-stage with the correct percept (the C-phase).

As a counterpart to leaking mechanisms, we have selected another sign of severe anxiety reported in Chapter 2 — *fusion*. To review: this term refers to phases in which the threat, or someone corresponding to the A_2 stimulus, draws close to the hero in B_2, climbs over the windowsill, exchanges heads with the hero, merges with him, or is substituted for him until everything is thoroughly confused. In these cases A_2 may be seen by the subject as a threatening face, an old person, or a parent, but it is not an object or a playmate of the same age as the hero. As in the case of leaking mechanisms, we shall examine how, in the PG process following the fusion phase, the subject manages to restore the distance between the threat and the hero, or, as we prefer to interpret it, to stave off the danger of losing his identity.

Subjects

As the reader may recall, subjects in the normal group were selected so as to make all age levels comparable with respect to sex and social background. There were 72 schoolchildren (7–15) and 55 preschoolers (see also Table 7.1).

Subjects in the clinical group considered here ranged from 4 to 16 years in age. There were 57 schoolchildren and eight pre-schoolers. In general, these children came from less academic families than did the normals. However, the balance with re-spect to cognitive maturity was approximately the same as in the normal group. While there were six immature children in a total of 33 in the age group (11)12–16 years (there were none in the normal group), there were only nine out of a total of 24 in the age group 7–10(11) (a distribution equivalent to the normal group).

Method

Afterimage Test

An AI series was considered to be intact if the child had been able to measure and describe AIs in at least eight trials. Children who lost more than two AIs (mostly the young and immature ones) will be dealt with below. Two scoring categories will be utilized here:

1. *Regressive instability:* There are shifts from normal AIs to childish ones, i.e., from a size ≥ 8.0 cm to a size ≤ 6.5 cm, from negative to positive color, or from an AI reflecting the form and meaning of the stimulus to an AI with a different, more concrete or physiognomic form and meaning. These changes may occur from one trial to a later one (with no more than two trials inter-vening) or within the same trial. Only in cases where the initial phase of the series is normal and no phases intervene between the normal and the primitive phase should regressions be considered to be true signs of psychotic discontinuity. (Two of the subjects in this study had such regressions.)

2. *Primitive series:* All AIs in the series are ≤ 6.5 cm, or all AIs are positive, or some AIs are positive and the rest are achromatic. The more cognitively mature a subject, the less likely he is to have entirely primitive AIs.

META-CONTRAST TECHNIQUE

The following main scoring categories will be considered here (a few more marginal categories are deferred to their proper context below). Most of these refer to the threat series, the exception being zero-phases, which were also scored in the car and room series.

Severe Anxiety

1. *Zero-phases:* At least two reports are given in which nothing or only chaos is perceived.

2. *Fusion:* This follows the description in Chapter 2, with particular care taken to avoid possible misunderstandings of the child's use of words.

3. *Leaking mechanisms:* This follows the description in Chapter 2, with an added differentiation between anxiety revealed in the percept and anxiety noted in the subject's behavior or thinking.

4. *Fright, etc.:* The child reports that he is frightened by the stimulus or openly expresses anxiety in other ways. (This sign was scored regardless of age. As is demonstrated below, however, it can hardly be considered a sign of severe anxiety in children too young for internalized reactions.)

5. *Hero disappears:* The child points out that the hero in B_2 has left the room, vanished, etc.

Less Severe Anxiety

1. *Dark structures:* These are added to the stimuli or decidedly emphasized in the report.

Primitive Defenses[1]

1. *Eye-shutting behavior:* The child shuts his eyes when presented with the stimulus, as if to shield himself or stave off danger.

2. *Sleep behavior:* The child yawns, talks about sleep, etc.

3. *Denial:* The child denies the existence of A_2 in a rather undifferentiated and blunt way ("No," "It's not there anymore," "I can't see the man").

Phobic Repression

This is one of the defensive strategies in which the threat appears to be decathected. While stimulus-near revisions of A_2 (a bust, a mask) are counted as primitive hysteric forms of repression, such stimulus-distant changes as objects, harmless animals, and trees are treated as phobic.

---

[1] These three signs were typical of the immature preschoolers in our normal sample, but had almost disappeared in the cognitively mature $5\frac{1}{2}$- to 6-year-olds.

Isolation/Negation
The child reports concealing surfaces or white fields instead of A_2 or negates A_2's threatening character. (For the validation of this sign as typical of obsessive-compulsive neurosis, see the sources cited in Chapter 1.)

CLINICAL SYMPTOMS

The clinical children were rated for the presence or absence of a number of symptoms. This rating, as noted in Chapter 4, was based on information from members of the clinical staff and was performed independently of the test scoring. The following *general* dimensions for anxiety have been described in Chapter 5 (see p. 104):

1. *Paroxysmal anxiety* (even slightly uncertain symptoms were considered here).
2. *Chronic anxiety.*
3. *Focused anxiety.*
4. *More diffuse anxiety reactions.*

In addition, several *specific* ratings concern us here:

1. *Phobic anxiety:* Fear of harmless animals, rooms, places, objects, etc. (i.e., fear of the present, not of the absent [Bowlby, 1973]).
2. *Varied reactions when frightened:* Flight, freezing, attack, crying.
3. *A generally passive attitude.*
4. *Denial of one's own anxiety.*

ANXIETY SIGNS IN THE MCT

Let us first present some validation data for leaking mechanisms, fusion, and other signs of severe anxiety. Table 7.1 reveals a clear difference between the clinical and the normal groups with respect to the frequency of signs of severe anxiety. For example, if we collapse the age groups and compare the normal and the clinical groups using the chi-square test, there is statistical support for the assertion that the clinical group showed severe anxiety signs more often ($\chi^2 = 25.70$, $df = 1$, $p < 0.005$, one-tailed). Fusion appears to be more typical of the young children

TABLE 7.1

SIGNS OF SEVERE ANXIETY IN CLINICAL AND NORMAL GROUPS

MCT Anxiety Signs	Clinical Group						Normal Group	
	Paroxysmal or chronic anxiety		Rest without paroxysmal or chronic anxiety		All clinical subjects			
	+	−	+	−	+	−	+	−
Zero-phases								
(11)12–16	5	16	0	12	5	28	0	36
7–10(11)	2	10	1	11	3	21	1	35
4–6	1	4	0	3	1	7	9	46
Fusion								
(11)12–16	5	16	2	10	7	26	0	36
7–10(11)	1	11	3	9	4	20	2	34
4–6	3	2	1	2	4	4	8	47
Leakage								
(11)12–16	9	12	6	6	15	18	3	33
7–10(11)	6	6	1	11	7	17	5	31
4–6	1	4	2	1	3	5	6	49
Fright								
(11)12–16	7	14	1	11	8	25	0	36
7–10(11)	4	8	0	12	4	20	0	36
4–6	2	3	1	2	3	5	9	46
Hero disappears								
(11)12–16	5	16	2	10	7	26	0	36
7–10(11)	4	8	2	10	6	18	0	36
4–6	1	4	2	1	3	5	13	42
Presence of sign								
(11)12–16	16	5	7	5	23	10	3	33
7–10(11)	10	2	6	6	16	8	8	28
4–6	4	1	3	0	7	1	27	28

and leaking mechanisms of the older ones. One of the signs, "hero disappears," is not uncommon among young preschool children and caution should be used in interpreting it as a sign of severe anxiety in these age groups. As expected, even such a strong sign as fright loses some of its power at the preschool level.

Table 7.2 compares the number of scored anxiety dimensions with symptomatic levels of anxiety in the clinical group of schoolchildren. Signs of severe anxiety clearly differentiate the clinically defined anxiety groups, whereas dark structures seem to differentiate between clinical and normal subjects at a more general level. If we contrast cases with paroxysmal and chronic anxiety, on the one hand, and the remaining clinical cases, on the other, with respect to the number of severe anxiety signs, we obtain a χ^2 (corrected for continuity) of 11.01 ($df = 3$, $p < 0.01$, one-tailed). A comparison between clinical and normal groups with respect to dark structures yields a χ^2 of 11.88 ($df = 1$, $p < 0.0005$, one-tailed).

TABLE 7.2

MCT ANXIETY SIGNS AND ANXIETY SYMPTOMS IN CLINICAL SCHOOLCHILDREN

Anxiety symptom rating	Number of severe anxiety dimensions in MCT				Dark structures	
	≥ 3	2	1	0	+	−
Paroxysmal	3	3	3	1	7	3
Chronic	5	3	11	6	14	11
Focused	1	1	5	6	11	2
Rest of sample	0	1	6	5	7	5
(Normals)					(26)	(46)

LEAKING MECHANISMS

Twenty-five subjects showed leaking mechanisms. If we focus on the PG process following the leaking phase, we find four subgroups.

1. *Regression:* After the leaking phase, the subject resorts to a more primitive defense, i.e., a defense typical of normal cognitively immature preschoolers. This subgroup included six patients, all of them of school age. In five of them, the leaking mechanism was of a compulsive type (isolation with a curtain, white spots in the window, or a denial-negation fraught with obvious compulsive qualities). In the remaining patient, we observed a phobic-repressive type of leaking mechanism. Five subjects resorted to eye-shutting behavior after the leaking

phase, while one applied a perceptual structure used in the first MCT series (a change shown to be analogous to regression, see Smith, Johnson, Ljunghill-Andersson, and Almgren, 1970).

2. *C-phase-follows:* The leaking phase leads to a correct report of A_2, without intervening incorrect reports. Of the seven patients in this group (six of them schoolchildren), one had a compulsive defense, one hero duplication (the threat was perceived as the hero's playmate), four phobic repression, and one stimulus-near repression. However, in five of these subjects the correct report was accompanied by attempts to walk away or to seek refuge with the experimenter, by evasive talk, pronounced yawning, or reports that the hero had disappeared in B_2.

3. *Reinforcement, or reinforcement with regression:* After the leaking phase, the subject repeats the same defense, but more emphatically. Four patients belonged to the pure reinforcement subgroup, two to the mixed subgroup. Five of them were schoolchildren. In one patient, the leaking mechanism was hero duplication (strengthened by making the duplicate the hero's twin) and, in the other five, more or less vaguely structured patterns (e.g., something in-between a hippie and a dog changing to a statue, or a cracked window later supplied with an extra pane).

4. *Nonregressive change:* After the leaking phase, the subject shifts to another mechanism, but not a primitive one. Of the six patients in this group (all schoolchildren), one changed from leaking hero duplication to phobic repression, two from phobic repression to isolation or reaction formation (A_2 reported as benevolent), and three from stimulus-near repression to isolation or isolation plus reaction formation.

MATURITY AND AI INSTABILITY

In further differentiating these four subgroups, we compared the cognitive maturity of the subjects in each (see Table 7.3). The following were considered signs of immaturity: preschool age, an "immature" score on the landscape test relative to the subject's age, and primitive AIs. A few of the subjects who could not or who refused to produce AIs belonged to the preschool group anyway.

To complete our picture of the regression subgroup, in particular, we also wished to consider regressive instability in the AI test. Only series that were intact (with at least eight measurements) were inspected. On finding that not only the regression subgroup but also the C-phase subgroup was characterized by AI instability, we decided to see if these two groups could be differentiated by means of clinical ratings. Here phobic symptoms were an obvious choice as a rating category in view of the many phobic mechanisms found in the MCT protocols of the C-phase subgroup. Passivity and attacking behavior were selected because of the contrasting primitive MCT defenses of the two subgroups: sleepiness versus more active warding off.

1. *Regression:* Three of the six patients showed some sign of cognitive immaturity. Further, five patients were scored for instability in the AI test. We have already pointed out that after the leaking phase their MCT protocols were characterized by primitive defensive strategies; looking at the full protocols, we find five patients with eye-shutting behavior and two with blunt denials. Only one child showed sleep behavior. On a clinical level, attacking behavior when frightened was noted in five (Table 7.4).

2. *C-phase follows:* Signs of cognitive immaturity were found in two of the seven patients. Yet four of the five patients with intact AI series were scored for instability. Unlike the regression subgroup, however, the primitive defense of eye-shutting behavior did not predominate (three of seven) and none of these patients exhibited denial. We noted above a number of passive-evasive reactions after the leaking phase. It is not surprising, then, to find that five subjects showed sleep behavior in their protocols; a sixth subject let the hero disappear from the picture. Clinically, four of these children were described as phobic and six as passive.

3. *Reinforcement:* As shown in Table 7.3, five of the six patients in this subgroup had at least one sign of cognitive immaturity. It should also be mentioned that in three patients anxiety was observed on the behavioral, rather than the perceptual, level.

4. *Nonregressive change:* As could have been expected, there were no signs of cognitive immaturity in these six patients. In all of them, anxiety was scored on the perceptual level. This

TABLE 7.3
LEAKING MECHANISMS AND MATURITY CRITERIA

Leaking subgroups	N	1 Preschool children	2 Cognitively immature school-children	3 Primitive AIs	4 Anxiety on behavioral level	Some sign 1–3	No sign 1–3
Regression	6	0	2	1	1	3	3
C-phase follows	7	1	1	1	2	2	5
Reinforcement	6	1	1	4	3	5	1
Nonregressive change	6	0	0	0	0	0	6
All with leakage, no fusion	17	1	1	3	3	5	12
All with fusion, no leakage	7	3	0	2	—	5	2

subgroup, then, is at the upper end of the maturity scale, with the reinforcement subgroup at the lower end; this difference is significant ($p = 0.004$, Fisher's exact test, two-tailed).

We shall now test the difference between the first two subgroups and the rest of the leaking patients in relation to regressive instability in the AI test. As revealed in Table 7.4 — where only intact series are given — nine of 11 children in the first two subgroups were scored for such regression but only one of 10 in the other subgroups was so scored ($p = 0.003$, Fisher's exact test, two-tailed). The difference in the presence of eye-shutting behavior or denial in five children in the regression subgroup and none in the C-phase subgroup proved significant ($p = 0.01$, Fisher's exact test, two-tailed). The contrast of one phobic MCT score in the regression subgroup against seven in the C-phase subgroup yielded the same p value. On the other hand, the observations of phobic symptoms were not significant. However, only five children in the entire group of 25 demonstrated clear phobic symptoms, four of them in the C-phase subgroup ($p = 0.025$, Fisher's exact test, two-tailed).

To summarize, the regression and C-phase subgroups differed from the other two subgroups on AI instability. The C-phase patients were more phobic than the regression ones and generally less inclined to use active warding-off strategies. The two AI-stable subgroups, reinforcement and nonregressive change, differed on cognitive maturity, with the latter subgroup being clearly more mature.

FUSION

Fifteen protocols were scored for fusion. The group as a whole is relatively immature, including most of the preschool children, as well as most of the cognitively immature schoolchildren, and many children with thoroughly primitive AIs. This trend was expected since older and cognitively-emotionally more mature subjects, with a clearer sense of self, would not allow fusion to happen.

It seemed more difficult to classify subjects within the fusion group than it was for the group with leaking mechanisms. One obvious reason was the smaller size of the group. Nevertheless,

TABLE 7.4

DESCRIPTION OF REGRESSION AND C-PHASE SUBGROUPS

Subgroup	AI Instability*		MCT Signs										Clinical Description					
			Eye shutting		Denial		Sleep		Eye shutting or denial, not sleep		Phobic repression		Attacking		Passive		Phobic	
	+	−	+	−	+	−	+	−	+	−	+	−	+	−	+	−	+	−
Regression	5	1	5	1	2	4	1	5	5	1	1	5	5	1	2	4	1	5
C-phase follows	4	1	3	4	0	7	5	2	0	7	7	0	3	4	6	1	4	3
Reinforcement and nonregressive change	1	9																

* Only complete series were scored.

a possible subdivision suggested itself. After the fusion phase, one subgroup of subjects tried to structure some sort of defense on the perceptual level, even a leaking defense. The other subjects did not show this defensive structuring. Instead, a C-phase might immediately follow the fusion; the PG process might move into zero-phases or phases openly expressing anxiety; or there might be impairment of the perceptual structure, sleep behavior, repeated denials, etc.

To characterize these two subgroups further, we focused on the child's way of reacting when frightened. We would expect the subjects who made some attempt at defensive structuring to be better able to face reality, while the others would be more resigned, more inclined to flee, and less capable of self-understanding (that is, of admitting their own anxieties). Three of the six patients with defensive structuring were immature according to our criteria, compared with seven of the nine patients in the other subgroup. Table 7.5 presents the findings on the behavioral characteristics chosen to distinguish between the two subgroups: crying, flight, freezing, and denial of anxiety. A significant difference between the two subgroups appears for freezing ($p = 0.012$, Fisher's exact test, two-tailed). If we consider the clinical signs 2–5 in Table 7.5 together, we see that in the defensive-structuring subgroup no child showed more than one sign, while in the other subgroup every child showed at least two signs ($p < 0.002$, Mann-Whitney, two-tailed).

Discussion

Our observation that at times children's defensive structures appear to "leak" anxiety agrees well with clinical findings. Anna Freud (1970), comparing children and adults, writes that children's "defensive moves against anxiety [are] more often incomplete, i.e., partly unsuccessful" (p. 177). This impression may be taken as indirect support for our test findings. More concretely, we tried to assess the validity of our observations by directly comparing the clinical group with a normal population and by differentiating between degrees of anxiety within the clinical group. With regard to the latter, we placed so-called

TABLE 7.5
DESCRIPTION OF FUSION SUBGROUPS

Subgroup	1 Immature signs		2 Crying		3 Flight		4 Freezing		5 Denial of anxiety		Σ 2-5	
	+	-	+	-	+	-	+	-	+	-	≥2	<2
Defensive structuring after fusion	3	3	2	4	1	5	0	6	2	4	0	6
No defensive structuring	7	2	7	2	6	3	7	2	5	4	9	0

paroxysmal anxiety at the top of our scale and diffuse anxiety reactions at the bottom.[2] Signs of leaking defenses were most closely related to paroxysmal anxiety and to chronic anxiety (the level just below).

In our validation study we also included a number of other anxiety signs. Of special interest is fusion of the threat and the hero. Fusion seems to reflect problems somewhat different from those reflected by leaking defenses — problems less related to specific categories of defense and more generally bound to violations of the child's sense of identity and basic security. It is therefore not surprising that signs of fusion were most typical of young or cognitively immature subjects. With both fusion and leaking mechanisms, our attention was mainly directed to how the child organized his defense in the PG phases following the one in which fusion or leaking mechanisms appeared (i.e., after the defensive strategy proved to be inefficient).

Before discussing our results in more detail, we would like to dwell briefly on the question of a defensive hierarchy from a developmental perspective. At the beginning of this chapter, we described how defensive regression could be operationally defined in the MCT: either in relation to the subject's own percept genesis or in relation to MCT data from children at various age and maturity levels. It should be noted that our findings agree well with most clinical accounts, in which, for instance, denial is seen as an early, narcissistic defense, while isolation, regression, and reaction formation are classified as later, neurotic mechanisms (Vaillant, 1971; see also A. Freud, 1936; Symonds, 1945; Fenichel, 1946; G. Bibring, Dwyer, Huntington, et al., 1961; Cameron, 1963; Kolb, 1968). With regard to the more "advanced" strategies, we follow Anna Freud (1970) and others who consider repression to be a less mature defense than isolation. The defensive strategies defined by the MCT might thus be ranked as follows (starting with the low-level narcissistic strategies): eye-shutting behavior, primitive denial, eye shutting by the hero, hero duplication (a strategy that still has narcissistic aspects), primitive repression, phobic

[2] It should be noted again here that Cameron (1963) considers paroxysmal anxiety to be a regression to primary anxiety, i.e., an irresistible need to discharge tension under any stress.

repression, isolation-negation/reaction formation.

We shall now turn to the specific analysis presented in this chapter.

LEAKING MECHANISMS

Leaking mechanisms were relatively easy to define and to spot in the protocols once the line between leaking and non-leaking mechanisms had been defined. Where exactly to draw this line does, naturally, remain to some degree a matter of personal choice. The subgroups we distinguished tended to overlap on certain criteria. Yet our sample was small; with more cases, a more nuanced differentiation should be possible. In any case, our classification showed some significant differences.

Let us first examine the split between the two unstable and the two stable subgroups. Regressive instability was defined by the AI data and referred to the sudden appearance of immature AIs among more mature ones. The AI results may seem a rather obscure and artificial measure for clarifying clinical differences. AI regressions have, however, proved to be valid and reliable signs of a subject's tendency to oscillate between more and less mature forms of reality adaptation (see Smith, Ruuth, Franzén, and Sjöholm, 1972). Moreover, given the empirically established difference between children and adults with respect to AI size and color, regressive instability can be clearly defined in operational terms.

Although in the MCT both AI-stable subgroups seem to be able to replace the leaking mechanisms with more effective strategies, without recourse to regression, they differ on the age-maturity scale. The *nonregressive-change* subgroup chooses more sophisticated strategies, shifting from hero duplication to phobic repression and from repression to isolation or reaction formation. In the *reinforcement* subgroup, the same defensive tactic is tried again, but the second time it is used more emphatically than in the leaking phase, where the attempt is often unfocused and hesitant. The relative immaturity of these children may explain the lack of "finality" in their initial defensive strategies, as well as their readiness to repeat them in spite of the first failure.

The two AI-unstable subgroups differ with respect to the kind of primitive defense used. After the leaking phase, the *regression* subgroup falls back on eye-shutting behavior or, in a few cases, active denial. Instead, the *C-phase* subgroup seems inclined to surrender in a passive manner by withdrawing in sleepiness (or, in one case, by simply letting the hero disappear). In this latter group the most common MCT mechanisms were phobic ones, i.e., mechanisms basically employing displacement and avoidance. The regression subgroup tended to show more compulsive patterns of defense. It did not regress halfway after the leakage but *all the way* to a primitive and probably less demanding level of functioning. In looking at the kinds of primitive strategies scored in the protocols of our "leaking" subjects — isolating-negating subjects, on the one hand, and phobic subjects, on the other — we may learn something about possible precursors of these defense mechanisms.

Fusion

The identification of fusion may have been a trifle more difficult than that of leaking mechanisms because the children with fusion were generally younger or cognitively more immature and therefore apt to use more ambiguous language. Even with respect to fusion, however, agreement between the judges of the protocols was practically 100%.

From the beginning, it was assumed that fusion would be a rather severe sign of anxiety, particularly prevalent in young and immature children. Fusion between the hero and the threat implies invasion of the child's person. An important aspect of cognitive and emotional development is the growing autonomy of the individual in relation to the world around him. As long as the differentiation between self and other remains vague or confused, the appearance of an unknown "other" is likely to be perceived as an intrusion on the "self" and, therefore, as a potential danger to the child's identity. This assumption seemed to be confirmed (see Table 7.1), even if the number of subjects was too small to allow definitive conclusions.

The difference between the two fusion subgroups is revealing. It appears that children lacking structured defensive alternatives to counteract the threat of fusion are more disturbed than children who can mobilize at least some kind of repressive or isolating effort, however inefficient. Apparently, the mere finding that internal defensive strategies have started to supersede the primitive external tactics is an important sign of ego maturity, i.e., of the child's ability to define his own self as something distinct from the outside world and to integrate his sense of self with his emotional and cognitive experiences.

Conclusion

Our study was designed to investigate, at the concrete perceptual level afforded by the MCT, the dilemmas confronting anxiety-ridden children and young adolescents. How do different children try to handle anxiety-provoking situations? Of particular import were inefficient defensive resources and an uncertain sense of self. We were able to define operationally one reason for defensive regression to low-level strategies — leaking mechanisms. We could also pinpoint what we assume to be a major obstacle to a child's normal emotional development — vulnerability to invasions into the "self region" of experience.

8

ANXIETY AND THE
META-CONTRAST TECHNIQUE

This chapter focuses on the MCT signs of anxiety in the clinical group. While a number of new findings will be presented, we also intend to integrate our data with findings reported in previous chapters. Let us first briefly review the results of our work with normal children and with selected clinical subjects. As we discussed in Chapter 2, in the absence of clinical criteria, results from the AI test were used as tentative measures of anxiety. The correlated strong or moderate MCT signs of anxiety appeared to be zero-phases, broken structures, and fusion. (Other signs of anxiety, such as impairment of defensive formations, dark structures, and hero discontinuity were presented in Chapter 2.[1])

We found some difference between prepubescent and pubescent subjects (12–15 years), on the one hand, and younger subjects, on the other. Given the greater instability of young children's perceptual reports, we had assumed that for them signs of structural impairment would be less indicative of anxiety than for the older children. The results appeared to confirm this hypothesis. A more common sign of anxiety in young subjects was hero discontinuity (reports of the hero walking out of the picture or simply disappearing). In addition, it was important to distinguish between early and late reports of dark structures, especially in the percept genesis of older children, as a late report was more indicative of *manifest,* as opposed to latent, anxiety.

[1] Fusion and leaking mechanisms, both common in our pilot group of anxiety-ridden children, were of particular importance for the clinical group. These signs have already been discussed in detail in Chapter 7.

When we extended our work with normal schoolchildren to preschool children (Chapter 3), it became more important than before to pay attention to the child's behavior in the testing situation. These very young children could not internalize the anxiety triggered by the MCT, but had to express it directly in their behavior. Even adults and older children sometimes openly exhibit anxiety when tested. In addition, we observed how young children tried to flee from the whole situation by walking away or running to the experimenter for comfort. Although these signs often suggested attempts at defense, they were obviously also expressions of direct anxiety because the defense afforded only momentary escape or relief. Preschool children also typically showed other "nonstructural" but more clear-cut defensive operations, such as eye-shutting behavior or outright denial of the existence of any threat. These manifestations, however, were considered to be *indirect* signs of imminent anxiety and are therefore not included in the present study of manifest anxiety.

SUBJECTS

Altogether there were 68 children (40 boys and 28 girls). Thirty-five were 12 years or older (or mature 11-year-olds). Among the remaining 33 younger children, eight were of preschool age.

RESULTS AND CONCLUSIONS

Given our previous findings, as well as the four classes of clinical anxiety (paroxysmal, chronic, focused, and more diffuse), we decided to arrange the MCT signs in a four-level hierarchy.

1. At the highest level we counted *openly expressed fright* in the testing situation (particularly, in schoolchildren where "internalized fright" would be a more normal reaction) and/or reports of *broken structures*. These signs were assumed to correspond to *paroxysmal anxiety*. It will be remembered that paroxysmal anxiety is

closely allied with feelings of impending disaster. This is one reason why reports of structures breaking down or dissolving were placed at this level of the hierarchy. In order to obtain a sufficient number of signs, we accepted slightly doubtful signs at this level (as we did in our clinical estimation of paroxysmal anxiety).

2. At a slightly lower level we placed other signs known to correspond to states of severe anxiety: *fusion* of the hero and the threat, *leaking mechanisms*, at least *two zero-phases* where nothing meaningful was perceived, direct attempts at *flight* from the testing situation. While the first three signs are more or less self-evident as indicators of severe, although not necessarily paroxysmal, anxiety, the inclusion of flight may appear debatable. It is not the same as panic since an attempt to escape is not completely unorganized. On the other hand, by fleeing the subject demonstrates his inability to master the anxiety provoked by the MCT. The placement of flight one step below panic seems right.

3. Here we find reports that the *hero has disappeared* (sheer neglect by the subject to mention the hero was not counted), that *human forms corresponding to* (but not implying correct identification of) A_2 *are impaired or missing;* and that *dark structures appear in the last third of the* $A + B$ *sequence* (correct but not unduly emphasized reports of blackness were not counted). The first sign represents escape; it is symbolic flight. Impairment of defensive structures has already been shown to correspond to clinical symptoms of anxiety. Human forms represent a rather advanced type of defense, close to the C-phase level; thus their impairment is a more manifest kind of anxiety than impairment of less advanced structures.[2] These signs, as well as the direct reflection of anxiety in darkness close to the C-phase, do not seem to be quite on a par with signs at level 2 but are more marked than signs at level 4.

4. The lowest level includes *nonhuman structures (corresponding to* A_2) *which are impaired or missing; dark structures before the last third of the* $A + B$ *sequence; diffuse formations* (fog, a rain-streaked or dirty window, etc.); *somatic signs* (a sudden need to go to the toilet, etc.); and *the subject's seeking shelter with the experimenter.* This collection is one of early, less advanced, or more indirect signs.

This classification of anxiety signs was supported by a comparison of the clinical subjects and normal subjects (Chapter 7). One group of signs was more or less exclusively concentrated in

---

[2] It should be noted that even if a structure is impaired, perceptual signs of anxiety do not "leak" through the defensive fabric, as is the case with leaking mechanisms.

the clinical group, at least at school age: open fright, zero-phases, fusion, and leaking mechanisms. Specifically, zero-phases were scored in 14% of the clinical schoolchildren and 1% of the normal ones. The other respective figures were: for fusion, 19% and 3%; for leaking, 37% and 11%; and for open fright, 21% and 0%. "Hero has disappeared" also clustered in the clinical schoolchildren (23%, compared with 0% in the normals), but this sign was more common than the others among normal preschool children (see also below). Black forms, regardless of placement, differentiated less clearly between anxiety-ridden schoolchildren (65%) and normal ones (36%). The flight sign could not be evaluated here because it had not been considered in testing the normal group.

Due to its relative scarcity, "broken structures" was also omitted from the above comparison. Looking into this now, we find that it was not completely absent from the normal group. However, if we limit our scoring to cases where the report of a broken structure also seems to reflect an impending dissolution of the ordinary world, the sign occurs only in the clinical subjects. Four clinical subjects showed this sign. Two of these four also displayed open fright. One of the two remaining cases expressed end-of-the-world fears. The remaining child only reported a broken window, but he repeated this description several times. We might have excluded him from the group with severe broken-structure signs. Moreover, his anxiety was not rated as paroxysmal. Nevertheless, we placed him among the severe cases in order not to favor our hypotheses unduly.

The different anxiety symptoms were unevenly distributed over age levels. Paroxysmal anxiety, in particular, was present in only one subject below the age of 12. (The younger a subject, the less deviant an outbreak of so-called primary anxiety would seem to be.) Because of this, we have represented older subjects separately in Table 8.1. On the whole, however, it does not make much difference whether comparisons are based on the entire group or only on subjects above 11 years of age.

The main trends in Table 8.1 are obvious; many were highly significant (see also Tables 7.1 and 7.2). In the left column, the level 1 MCT signs are concentrated in the paroxysmal group. Level 2 signs are also slightly more typical of this group. A bet-

TABLE 8.1
OVERVIEW OF HIERARCHY OF MCT ANXIETY SIGNS AND CLINICAL ANXIETY SYMPTOMS

Clinical Anxiety Rating	MCT Signs											
	Level 1		Level 2		Level 1+2		Level 3		Level 4		N
	≥1 sign	%	≥1 sign	%	≥2 signs	%	≥1 sign	%	≥1 sign	%	
Paroxysmal											
(11)12–16	7		7		6		7		7		9
All	8	80	7	70	6	60	7	70	7	70	10
Chronic											
(11)12–16	2		7		4		8		8		13
All	8	27	19	63	9	30	21	70	16	53	30
Focused											
(11)12–16	0		6		1		8		3		8
All	0	0	8	62	2	15	12	92	4	31	13
Diffuse											
(11)12–16	1		2		1		4		2		5
All	2	13	6	40	2	13	9	60	6	40	15

ter differentiation between all four anxiety groups is afforded by the third column, in which levels 1 and 2 are combined. The great number of level 3 signs in the group with focused anxiety will be analyzed in more detail later. At the lowest symptom level, it can be observed that the percentage of MCT signs is relatively low at level 1 and reaches a peak at level 3. The fact that subjects with high-level signs were also scored for lower-level signs is consistent with the fact that severe clinical symptoms are often combined with less severe ones.

The group of clinical subjects presented in Table 8.1 does not shed full light on the age differences between the various signs. In Chapter 7, however, we demonstrated that fusion appeared in young or cognitively immature subjects and leaking in older or more mature ones. The probability of experiencing intrusion from the outside was deemed to be particularly high in children in whom the sense of self was not yet clearly articulated. Similarly, leaking should not only be more easily noticed in subjects with well-structured defenses but should also represent a more serious alarm signal.

Chapter 7 also indicated that "hero has disappeared" did not differentiate between normal and clinical subjects as effectively as fusion and leaking. To be more precise, this relative lack of differentiating power occurred at the preschool level, where 24% of the normals had this sign. However, even if the sign does differentiate well between normal and clinical schoolchildren, there are no convincing indications within the clinical group that it is on a par with level 2 signs. One more result deserves to be cited here: no normal schoolchildren were scored for open fright, but 16% of the preschool children received this score. Again, we had expected that this sign would lose its power as the subjects decreased in age.

We also assumed that zero-phases would be typically related to age and cognitive maturity. The more unstable a child's conception of outside reality, the less indicative of anxiety these intermittent breaks in a series of perceptual reports would be. This hypothesis was supported by Chapters 2 and 3 but could not be clearly confirmed here, as the sign was not particularly common. It may be surmised that our increased reluctance to score zero-phases as the age of the subjects decreased contributed to making zero-phases appear more equal diagnostically at different age levels. This may also have been true of "flight," which did not, as expected, become "less severe" as the age of the subjects decreased.

As far as level 1 signs among 12- to 16-year-old subjects are concerned, we would like to emphasize not only their correlation with paroxysmal anxiety but also with other signs of serious dysfunctioning. In Chapter 5 we showed that AI discontinuity coincided both with paroxysmal symptoms and level 1 MCT anxiety signs *and* with signs of discontinuity in the PG process laid bare by the MCT. Among these discontinuities were zero-phases. A sudden break in the stable frame percept is thus likely to indicate two conditions: discontinuous (often near-psychotic or psychotic) functioning and spells of severe anxiety. As seen in Table 8.1, zero-phases and other level 2 signs may be indicative of paroxysmal forms of anxiety, but less exclusively than level 1 signs.

One difference indicated in Table 8.1 is that children with chronic anxiety had several types of severe signs while those with focused anxiety usually showed fewer signs. Above all, children with focused anxiety lacked signs of open fright; in line with their phobic and pseudo-phobic fears, they appear particularly inclined to project anxiety into reports of dark perceptual formations. Of 13 focused-anxiety subjects, 11 reported blackness but no level 1 signs; of 30 chronic subjects, only 13 made such a report ($p = 0.02$, Fisher's exact test, two-tailed), and 13 did not report blackness at all.

We have reason to assume that our anxiety dimensions can be applied to older subjects. Previous studies of anxiety-ridden adults yield comparable data, particularly from adolescents. Even the brain-injured subjects excluded from our group of children substantiate observations made in adults: all subjects with brain dysfunction are characterized by their inability to bring structure to the tachistoscopic material, at least until exposure times have been prolonged far beyond the normal length.

In placing anxiety signs within a hierarchy, we would caution the reader (and ourselves as well) against relying too heavily on such a scoring scheme. The severity of a sign depends not only on its place in a diagnostic hierarchy but also on the context in which it appears. Thus, there is a difference between a subject in whom leaking leads to a subsequent strengthening of the defensive effort and one who responds with regression to infantile strategies or who submits to direct flight (the latter case would probably have a more negative prognosis). Similarly, fusion is a more serious indication in a person lacking structured defenses than in someone who reveals the availability of such defenses in his percept genesis.

In addition, the position of a sign, late or early, may be important. Only black features were differentiated here with respect to position, mainly because most severe signs appeared at comparatively late trials in the PG process anyway. It should also be recognized that in young children a differentiation of early and late appearance could not always be made with certainty because of the indeterminateness of their C-phases.

In summary, then, the anxiety signs in the MCT should be considered in relation not only to age but also to their PG context. Mechanical recording is of little value and may lead to erroneous conclusions. Used with discrimination and a reasonable amount of psychological understanding, the MCT can serve to elucidate the role of anxiety in the context of an individual's adaptive and defensive endeavors.

9

STATISTICAL OVERVIEW OF
CLINICAL GROUP

Much of the information available from the clinical group has not yet been fully analyzed. Each subject was scored on 196 items for test signs and clinical symptoms (including age and cognitive maturity). Many of these scores are naturally bound to be sifted out because of relative scarcity. But the remaining items will certainly allow us to illuminate the clinical problem area in a more comprehensive way than before. The results presented in previous chapters are expected to facilitate this endeavor. What we shall thus attempt to do in summarizing the clinical part of our project is to give some order to the nonorganic mental disorders reflected in our sample of 57 schoolchildren, all of whom showed anxiety in some form and degree.

To group our empirical data, we plan to use an inverted factor analysis based on the G-index of agreement (Holley and Guilford, 1964). While a conventional factor analysis aims at grouping the variables (test scores, observations, estimates), an inverted factor analysis aims at grouping the individuals. We therefore use the term "person factors" here. A varimax rotation will result in a first factor solution, where the discriminating power of individual items can be tested by means of a special D-estimate (Holley and Risberg, 1972). Two alternative solutions will also be tried: one placing special weight on items pertaining to discontinuity in the test serials, paroxysmal anxiety, and other severe symptoms together with the contrast between older and younger age groups, and another stressing projective mechanisms and hypersensitivity (again in combination with age). These "natural" factor groupings will be supplemented by

163

a more systematic regrouping of the first factor solution.

Let us first summarize the three problem clusters on which we hope to throw some light: (1) the degree to which test items and behavior items (symptoms) associate in building the person factors; (2) the meaning of some intricate and central test signs, among them signs of projection which have not been treated in the preceding clinical chapters; (3) certain clinical issues such as psychotic manifestations at different age levels, the borderline personality in adolescence, the asymmetry of various developmental lines in the disturbed child, and the difference between reactive and structural disorders. The necessary prerequisite for the discussion of these and related questions is that they be reflected in sufficiently large and pronounced person factors.

Subjects

Since we had only eight subjects in the age range 4 to 6 years, we decided to focus on children 7 to 16 years of age. Of our 57 subjects, 13 (nine boys, four girls) were 7 to 8 years old, 14 (10 boys, four girls) were 9 to 11 years, 10 (four boys, six girls) were 12 to 13 years, and 20 (12 boys, eight girls) were 14 to 16 years. The reasons for excluding some of our original 7- to 16-year-old subjects were insufficient clinical or experimental data. Considering the obstacles we faced in testing psychiatrically disturbed youngsters, the loss of subjects was small.

Clinical Symptoms

Table 9.1 presents an overview of the distribution of some important symptom dimensions. Dimensions 1–4 are highly intercorrelated. When 4 is scored 5 is always scored also; 10 is included in 9. It is obvious that severe disturbances are more common or more easily identifiable among the older children. The young ones are more often characterized by depression and by more diffuse disturbances, which are difficult to categorize.

The uneven distribution of some symptoms may to some extent be caused by uneven sampling. Although our group probably represents a good sampling of the nonorganic cases at the

TABLE 9.1
DISTRIBUTION OF SOME SYMPTOM DIMENSIONS

Symptom	Percentage positive scores	
	7-11 years	12-16 years
1. Near-psychotic or psychotic reactions	4	17
2. Disturbed reality contact	4	37
3. Anticipations of disaster	7	20
4. Paroxysmal anxiety	4	27
5. Chronic anxiety	44	70
6. Outright separation anxiety	15	27
7. Attacking when frightened	41	53
8. Freezing when frightened	41	60
9. Depression	63	60
10. Depression without mania or compulsive rituals	41	27
11. Compulsive rituals	19	27

clinic, these cases do not necessarily reflect the general distribution of mental disturbances in children 7 to 16 years of age. It would be very surprising, however, if the distribution differences in Table 9.1 were not primarily caused by *true* developmental differences. To account for age, we have particularly stressed this dimension in factoring alternatives 2 and 3 below but have also included it in alternative 1.

As we have already shown in previous chapters, there are also frequency differences between age groups with respect to test signs, differences that often go with differences in cognitive maturity. These age differences, however, do not make it impossible to draw certain conclusions regarding the differential validity of test scores. Nevertheless, if "psychotic" signs are scored in the test protocols of our youngsters, but no psychotic symptoms appear, these signs are clearly not valid as signs of psychosis at that age level.

SCORING DIMENSIONS

A detailed description of the scoring dimensions seems unnecessary for our purposes here. We thus present only a brief outline grouping the dimensions with regard to the states and functions they represent: anxiety, depression, neurotic defense, psychosis, etc. Some of the dimensions have already been presented in previous chapters. Supplementary descriptions of key dimensions will be offered in due course.

AFTERIMAGE TEST

Originally there were 34 scoring dimensions pertaining to *primitive signs* (positive and/or size-constant AIs, etc.), *anxiety* (large and/or very dark AIs, five or more primitive AIs in children over 11 years of age, loss of more than two AIs, etc.), *process discontinuities* (abrupt shifts from normal to primitive AIs), *hypersensitivity* (variegated AIs), and *depressive retardation* (negative size regression over the AI serial). For details of these dimensions, see Chapter 5 and the factor analysis results below.

META-CONTRAST TECHNIQUE

Originally there were 107 scoring dimensions pertaining to *direct denial and avoidance* (the child shuts his eyes, starts to leave the test room, etc.), *narcissistic projection* (reports of a duplicate of the hero in the window), *severe anxiety* (signs of open fright in the test situation, reports of fusion between the hero and the threat, "leaking," broken structures, etc.), *moderate anxiety* (reports of diffuse or weakened defensive structures, of black structures, etc.), *projection* (extra persons or animals in B, other changes in B disrupting its identity, reports of movement), *hypersensitivity* (changes in B not affecting the subject's recognition of it), *process discontinuities* (zero-phases, i.e., B_2 suddenly reported as nonexistent, meaningless, etc.), *changes in the identification figure* (hero older, sadder, injured, etc.), *depressive retardation* (unbroken series of at least five incorrect and unchanged reports of A_2), *isolation* (a curtain, white screen, etc., in the window preventing the identification of A_2), *primitive repression* (only torn-off parts of A_2 reported), *hysteroid repression* (A_2 reported as a stiff statue, etc.), *phobic repression* (reports of a lifeless but more stimulus-distant A_2, e.g., an object). For details about these dimensions, see Smith, Sjöholm, and Nielzén (1975, 1976), previous chapters, and the factor analysis results below.

FACTOR ANALYSIS METHOD

As noted above, the inverted factor analysis (with varimax rotation and factor extraction down to Eigenvalues of 1.0) was based on the G-index of agreement developed by Holley and Guilford (1964), among others. This technique is particularly useful for the organization of clinical data with a dichotomous scoring provided that the number of persons is comparatively small and the number of items several times larger.

The 57 subjects were rated on 196 dimensions. One prerequisite for this kind of analysis is that an item be scored as present or absent in at least 10% of the sample. Mostly because of relative scarcity, the number of items in alternative 1 was reduced to six for age and cognitive maturity, 25 for the AI test, 64 for the MCT, and 45 for the clinical criteria—in all, 140 items. The number of items is thus relatively small in relation to the number of persons. In alternative 2 (focusing on discontinuities and severe symptoms), 18 items were repeated five times each, and in alternative 3 (emphasizing projection and hypersensitivity), nine items were repeated in the same way.

The person factors were identified as follows: only factor loadings ≥ 0.45 were accepted if, at the same time, the distance between the highest and the next highest loading was ≥ 0.10. In the majority of cases, loadings were considerably higher and distances greater.

When a factor solution had been decided on, a D-estimate of discrimination was calculated for each individual item. D is a simple measure of how much the item discriminated between the group of persons in a factor and all other persons in the sample (Holley and Risberg, 1972). The size of D is not independent of the size of the factor. There is no simple rule of thumb for the use of this estimate and no method for calculating its statistical significance. According to a very conservative rule, values of D < 0.50 are not worth considering, not even in factors of more than three persons. In small factors, we have tried to disregard values of D < 0.60 as far as possible. In the case of very small factors, we at times refer to alternative solutions where the same subjects are included among others in a larger factor.

The factors are numbered (with Roman numerals) in the order in which they appear in the rotated factor matrix. We discuss them in this order, except for factors with only two subjects, which are examined at the end and designated by Arabic numerals. Naturally, factors not meeting the statistical criteria just mentioned will not be discussed.

We have also tried an artificial "factor" solution. Using alternative 1 as a matrix, we have regrouped the subjects in order to systematically organize some important factor differences. D-estimates have been calculated in the usual fashion. Parts of this solution will be described together with Factor I_1, and Factor 9_2.[1]

Factor Analysis Results

Alternative 1

Ten factors encompassing 38 children will be considered in this solution; some of these are discussed only briefly. Most test signs and clinical symptoms characterizing the various factors have been presented in the scoring categories. In some instances, however, where the meaning of an item may still seem obscure, a more detailed description will be added here. D-values are shown within parentheses.

Factor I_1 (six subjects, including one under age 11 and four age 14 or older)

The sign that discriminates best (0.63) is size-constant AIs throughout the test series, a remarkable sign considering the age of most subjects. Clinically they are distinguished by non-diffuse anxiety symptoms (0.55).

---

[1] The subscripts refer to the particular alternative: i.e., Factor I (alternative 1) and Factor 9 (alternative 2).

Five of these subjects are also included in Factor I_3, where flight and freezing at frightening stimuli are typical reactions. This factor is, however, made up of six additional subjects. In the artificial factor solution, we have gathered seven subjects (four of them from Factor I_1) defined by age over 11 years, totally primitive AIs, and lack of the strongest anxiety sign in the MCT ("direct flight"). This group did not share any typical clinical symptoms.

In Chapter 5, we showed that adolescent subjects with permanent AI regression differ from subjects with intermittent regressions in not showing clear psychotic or near-psychotic symptoms, including signs of paroxysmal anxiety. These teenagers obviously react to anxiety with more or less permanent regression. Taken literally, AI regression implies an inability to distinguish between subjective and nonsubjective phenomena. We would expect this to be associated with a reduced capacity to identify with another person's perspective. The most extreme cases in the regression group conveyed an unmistakable impression of this "borderline" characteristic. The permanent regression — reflected in flight and freezing responses at the behavioral level — may offer a convenient escape route from more than temporary psychotic invasions. As we know, borderline cases are defined as not being permanently psychotic. The borderline symptom profile is also a vague and changing one — as in our subjects (see the discussion).

Factor III₁ (three subjects, age 9–13)

These children are distinguished by a long series of test signs. The most discriminating are: hero disappearance (0.83), an old A_2 (0.78), emphasis on the threat's eyes (0.87), hero duplication (0.69), and leaking mechanisms (0.69). There are no primitive AIs (0.63). The most important clinical symptom is situational anxiety (0.67).

Situational anxiety can be more concretely described as worry or anxious concern about one's own thoughts and acts in certain situations. These worries are associated with guilt feelings. The child's special interest in the eyes of an elderly A_2 in the window, for instance, probably reflects internalized demands from parents or other persons in authority (i.e., superego functions).

The intellectually well-equipped and cognitively mature children gathered under this factor had all been referred for "brief" psychotherapy, which we take as an indirect confirmation of their neurotic status. Yet their anxiety signs in the MCT — above all the tendency of their defenses to be inefficient — suggest that their neurotic disturbances are neither superficial nor easily cured.

Factor VI₁ (six subjects, age 14–16)

The AIs of this group are not primitive (0.67). In spite of this, they show eye shutting by the hero in the MCT (0.67). Their anxiety is described as diffuse (0.57) but as also having phobic characteristics (0.55). When frightened, they do not become aggressive (0.53).

There seems to be a contradiction in these subjects between a cognitively mature self-concept (the AI results) and a childishly evasive attitude toward the threatening stimulus. The emphatically nonaggressive behavior of these youngsters appears to reflect both cognitive maturity and emotional immaturity at one and the same time. This ambiguity may well explain some of the worry and uncertainty expressed by therapists concerning these patients (see the discussion).

Factor VII₁ (three subjects, age 9–16)

Two of these subjects are also included in Factor 5₃, where their severe disturbances stand out more prominently. We refer to the description of that factor.

Factor X₁ (four subjects, age 7–16)

Clinically, this group is clearly depressed, without any trace of mania or compulsive rituals (0.72). Three of the subjects reappear among the five subjects in Factor III₂, a factor with similar but more distinct characteristics.

Factor XI₁ (five subjects, age 7–13, three of them cognitively immature)

The factor is dominated by hero duplication continuing into late trials (0.81); given the immaturity of some of these subjects, this sign represents a relatively adequate narcissistic type of defense. In some cases, the hero duplication is combined with depressive stereotypy, i.e., the duplicate report is repeated in one trial after another without change (0.56). Paroxysmal and chronic anxiety are not noted (0.64), but instead more diffuse signs of anxiety are found (0.56). Characteristic of this not too seriously disturbed group is a stressful family background.

Factor XII₁ (five subjects, age 7–13)

These children's AI serials are clearly discontinuous (0.65). Clinically, three or even four of them can be regarded as seriously disturbed. Only among the older subjects, however, do the regressive AI signs appear to represent major breakthroughs of primitive functioning. Since regressions can reflect different steps on a child's developmental ladder and thus carry very different meanings at various stages, the lack of distinguishing symptoms in this factor is quite understandable.

Factor 4₁ (two subjects, ages 13 and 15)

The sign that differentiates best is five or more primitive AI phases in subjects over 11 years old (0.80). There seems to be no need to dwell on this small factor.

Factor 8₁ (two subjects, ages 8 and 12)

The following items in the MCT should be mentioned: hero disappearance (0.82); somatic signs, such as a sudden urge to go to the toilet (0.78); impairment from one trial to the next of nonhuman interpretations of the threat (0.80). Subjects also show sleepiness in the MCT situation (0.67) or try to divert the experimenter's attention from the task (0.66). The most typical clinical symptoms are nightmares (0.80). The subjects are anxiety-ridden and evasive at the same time. They try to talk themselves out of pressing problems, but their anxiety manifests itself in dreams or somatic symptoms.

Factor 9₁ (two subjects, both age 8, but cognitively mature for their age)

Here one notices motor unrest in the MCT (0.73), impairment from one trial to the next of defensive interpretations (0.84), depressive stereotypy (0.71), and direct denial of the threat (0.87). The dominant clinical signs are compulsions and rituals (0.80) combined with depression (0.76).

The compulsive components are perhaps the most striking features in this factor, at least if the young age is taken into account. Since the subsequent development of these children has been positive, one is tempted to assume that the compulsive defenses played a temporary but important role in guarding against severe regressions. In Factor X_2, which includes these two subjects and one other, hyperactivity is an additional characteristic (0.67), a symptom likely to be prognostically favorable in combination with childhood depression.

ALTERNATIVE 2

In this factor analysis the following items were assigned a weight five times that of other items:

1. *Age 7-11.*
2. *Five or more primitive AIs in children over 11 years old.*
3. *All AIs ≤ 6.5 cm* (i.e., practically size-constant).
4. *All AIs positive or achromatic* (i.e., primitive on a dimension other than size).
5. *Real AI regressions* (i.e., change from a phase with an adult AI to the next phase with a primitive one).
6. *AI depression* as described above.
7. Some anxiety-indicative *fusion* between the hero and the threat. One or more, or, alternatively, two or more *zero-phases.*
8. *Reports of open fear in the MCT* (even slightly marginal reports — one of the strongest anxiety signs in children not too young for internalized reactions).
9. *Depressive stereotypy.*
10. *Leaking mechanisms* (i.e., reports of a defensively disguised A_2 where the threatening qualities of A_2 are still coming to the fore).
11. *Leaking behavior* (where in an analogous way the child's behavior reveals the anxiety).
12. *Paroxysmal anxiety* (i.e., direct and sudden outbreaks of anxiety as described by Anthony [1975a], including even marginal cases — the irresistible need to discharge tension under any stress [Cameron, 1963] is a particularly serious symptom in the 12- to 16-year-olds, in whom it was most often scored).
13. *Paroxysmal anxiety or at least severe chronic anxiety.*
14. *Near-psychotic reactions of various kinds.*

15. *Cognitive disturbances* pertaining to the subject's contact with reality.

16. *Pervasive depressive mood* (devoid of all manic and compulsive components).

As must be obvious, we have particularly stressed items associated with discontinuities in the adaptive process, regressions to a primitive level of functioning, acute signs and symptoms of paroxysmal or at least very severe anxiety, psychotic or near-psychotic symptoms together with depressive signs and symptoms. These items, reflecting severe disturbances, were at times "hidden" among all the other, less severe signs in the first factor analysis.

Nine factors covering 39 subjects will be considered, only one of them at some length.

Factor I_1 (seven subjects, age 7–16, four cognitively immature for their age)

The highest D-value is noted for absence of paroxysmal or chronic anxiety (0.66). The group is characterized by diffuse anxiety and depression. The factor has three subjects in common with Factor XI_1.

Factor III_2 (five subjects, all age 10 or under)

These children have no AIs or truncated AI serials (0.78) and are inclined to run to the experimenter for shelter in the MCT situation (0.76). The clinical symptoms are regressive (0.62) but above all depressive, without manic or compulsive components (0.73).

Of the four subjects in Factor X_1, three reappear in this factor. The regressive and shelter-seeking tendencies add to the characterization of this depressive group. At the same time, the group cannot be considered seriously disturbed. These unhappy young children, who come from stressful homes, have reacted to their hardships with regressive wishes. We find no structural defects of any importance in this group.

Factor IV_2 (four subjects, three of them age 14–16)

The most distinguishing clinical symptom is paroxysmal anxiety (0.91), followed by disturbed reality contact (0.85) and near-psychotic reactions of other kinds (0.70) together with feelings of impending disaster (0.66). In the MCT open fright is most typical (0.62). The anxiety generated by the test is not bound in black structures (0.51). At least two AIs are positive (0.56).

This is a presumptive psychosis factor, where the paroxysmal anxiety is a serious core characteristic, particularly if regarded in relation to the subjects' older age. We shall return to these subjects when the artificial factor solution is presented in combination with Factor 9_2.

Factor V_2 (six subjects, all age 10 or under)

AI regression (0.70) cannot be considered a particularly noteworthy sign in these young and often cognitively immature subjects.

Factor VII_2 (three subjects, all over age 11)

The sign that distinguishes best is zero-phases in the MCT (0.83). Also noteworthy in regard to the subjects' age are the totally childish AIs (0.54). These children fear their own thoughts and fantasies (0.74), worry that they have been dangerously contaminated and are dying (0.72), and react with flight or freezing when frightened (0.52).

Two of these subjects are included in the six subjects in Factor I_1, a factor indicating borderline pathology with permanent AI regression (0.63). In the present selection of subjects the discontinuities in their percept genesis become more prominent.

Factor X_2 (three subjects, age 7–8)

The signs differentiating best are motor unrest in the MCT (0.74) and depressive stereotypy (0.72). Other characteristics are leaking behavior (0.59), denial (0.54), and reports of movement in the MCT (0.59). The clinical observations include hyperactivity (0.67) and attacking behavior when frightened (0.56).

Two of these children are grouped in Factor 9_1. We refer to the interpretation offered there, but also wish to point out the addition of leaking behavior (a primitive variant of leaking mechanisms). Although these children eventually solved their problems satisfactorily, they seem basically quite vulnerable.

Factor XII_2 (seven subjects, all over age 11, four of them age 14–16)

Reports of eye shutting by the hero (0.55) and flight (0.55) are characteristically immature defensive strategies for this age, and they contrast with the AI results (not even two positive or size-constant AIs [0.68]).

Factor 6₂ (two subjects, ages 12 and 13)

The most characteristic signs are leaking behavior (0.93), open fright in the MCT situation (0.86), hero disappearance (0.82), impairment of defensive structures (0.80), and five or more primitive AIs (0.80). Repression (A_2 is reported as an object) obtains a D of 0.84. Central clinical symptoms are hyperactivity (0.66), attacking behavior when frightened (0.55), and denial of anxiety (0.56).

Severe test anxiety appears in this group. The repressive strategies leak and cannot always contain the anxiety; the subject then reacts with more childish strategies and, at the behavioral level, with aggressive denial of the anxiety. (Cf. Factor 8_1.)

Factor 9₂ (two subjects, ages 10 and 15)

The following signs should be particularly noted: unstable (0.80) and variegated (0.78) AIs with clear discontinuities (0.82), fusion between the hero and the threat in the MCT (0.82), regressions to discarded interpretations (0.84), somatic reactions (0.78), tendencies to isolate the hero from the threat (0.75), and reports of movement (0.93). In the clinical picture we find fear that others will be contaminated or die (0.91) and also compulsive rituals.

The age difference between the two subjects explains why the regressive test signs have no clear counterparts in the symptom profile. Considering the present factor as well as Factor IV_2, we would like to present the artificial factor solutions.

Artificial Factors

Both of the artificial factors are defined by some discontinuity on the AI test and/or the MCT plus some sign of severe anxiety such as fusion, reports of broken structures, open fright, or leaking mechanisms. Factor A is also distinguished by an age of 12–16 years and by lack of permanent AI regression (see the discussion of this particular quality under Factor I_1). Factor B covers the age 7–11 years. For Factor A, we have also accepted cases showing open fright plus some other severe anxiety sign instead of discontinuity. With Factor B, this extra qualification would not have added any new subjects; it would not, moreover, have meant the same thing in this group of younger children.

Factor A includes six subjects. The central clinical symptom is paroxysmal anxiety (0.94). Other symptoms are disturbed reality contact (0.70) and near-psychotic reactions of other kinds (0.63). The signs chosen by us to characterize this group clearly represent psychotic symptoms in this group of older subjects.

This association is less clear in *Factor B* with its four subjects. Regression is the only clinical symptom worth mentioning (0.56). One might speculate about the lack of validity of these signs in younger age groups, a speculation wholly in line with our previous assumptions (cf. Factor XII_1). However, it should also be observed that the test signs chosen to distinguish the group are associated with phobic repression (0.62) and compulsive isolation (0.51) in the MCT protocols, defense mechanisms which evidently tend to keep outbreaks of anxiety in check.

ALTERNATIVE 3

In this factor analysis the following items were assigned a weight five times that of other items:

1. *Age 7–11.*
2. *Variegated AIs* (i.e., AIs shown to reflect hypersensitivity).
3. *Extra persons reported in one or both MCT series,* irrespective of previous correct reports of B.
4. *Extra animals* (instead of persons).
5. Reports of extra persons or extra animals preceded by a totally correct report of B.
6. *Subtle B changes* at least once (or at least twice in more marginal cases), i.e., changes in perspective, lighting, etc., which do not in any way endanger the identity of B to the observer.
7. *More drastic changes in B.*
8. Reports of *movement* in the MCT.

Here we have tried to emphasize the area of hypersensitivity-projection, partly because it had been overlooked in the previous clinical chapters in spite of its intrinsic interest. Most of these signs, however, had already been noted in the very first use of the MCT with clinical subjects (Smith and Henriksson, 1956).

Six factors involving 36 subjects are considered here, half of them only very briefly.

Factor I₃ (11 subjects, all over age 11)

Flight and freezing when frightened (0.61) are the clinical symptoms that discriminate best. Of six subjects in Factor I_1, five are included here. We refer to the description of that factor.

Factor II₃ (11 subjects, age 7–10)

This factor seems to have been determined mostly by age.

Factor III₃ (six subjects, age 7–15)

The AIs in this group are variegated (0.66) but tend to be negative (0.55). Extra persons are reported in the MCT series, either preceded by a correct C-phase (0.81) or not (0.98). There are also regressions in the MCT (0.53). The subjects are inclined to deny their anxiety (0.61).

Denial of anxiety and projection are probably two sides of the same coin. Still, the factor seems difficult to interpret. Extra persons are considered to be relatively serious signs in adolescence, while variegated AIs are often found in normal subjects, of all ages. The impression of the individual subjects in this factor is, however, that some of the older ones belong to our most disturbed cases. At any rate, these subjects are all hypersensitive-projective and hence bound to be vulnerable.

Factor IV₃ (four subjects, over age 11)

The presence of variegated AIs (0.81) goes together with subtle changes in the subjects' impression of B in the MCT (0.83). These subjects tend to separate A and B temporally before recognizing A (0.68). Typical clinical signs are nightmares (0.56) and attacking behavior when frightened (0.57). Sensitiveness is most typical of these subjects. This can be a favorable prognostic sign — which may also be true of their aggression.

Factor 5₃ (two subjects, age 11 and 15)

We have already discussed these subjects in conjunction with Factor VII_1. Here some characteristics are particularly accentuated: fusion between the hero and the threat (0.89), clear zero-phases (0.82), isolation tendencies (0.75), and denial of anxiety (0.56). On top of this there is projection of extra animals, even when preceded by a correct B (0.95).

Denial of anxiety and projection still belong together. However, a depressive tendency reflected in cumulative inhibition of AI size is added in this factor (0.69), as well as tendencies to isolation. In spite of their denial, these subjects are severe cases (see the discussion).

Factor 6₃

This factor is identical with Factor 9_2.

DISCUSSION

The association between test items and clinical symptoms is good. Most factors are determined by both kinds of items in combination. In a few instances, test signs do not seem to correlate with the expected clinical criteria in a factor description, but this does not necessarily mean that these signs lack validity. Depressive test signs and clinical signs of depression, for instance, do not always appear together in spite of the fact that their intercorrelation is very high indeed (Chapter 6). The reason for this may be, among other things, that the D-value of one of these items is just above the demarcation line chosen for the presentation of D-indices and the other just below. However, the joint occurrence of test items and criteria will be taken here to mean that, on the whole, our instruments reflect the clinical symptoms chosen to represent these children.

In discussing the test signs, we would like to begin with *emphasis on eyes* in descriptions of A_2. In adults, reference to eyes has been associated with projective strategies (Smith, Johnson, Ljunghill-Andersson, and Almgren, 1970). Here we find eye reports in Factor III_1, a group of subjects in the middle age range characterized by situational anxiety and feelings of guilt about their own thoughts and acts. Without speculating too much about the developmental roots of adult projection, we do not find it difficult to link children's preoccupation with their own thoughts and fantasies with an adult propensity for projecting this concern on the outside world. This link is made all the more probable by the fact that the children in this factor are intellectually well equipped and cognitively mature, while their disturbances seem to be more serious than appears at first sight.

It was shown in Chapter 2 that such signs of *projection in the MCT* as extra persons and animals in B are quite common at preschool age but tend to diminish as children grow older. We therefore wished to explore whether such signs would appear in older age groups among the present clinical subjects. Factors III_3, IV_3, and 5_3 are all characterized by hypersensitive-projective signs. In Factors III_3 and IV_3, these signs do not seem necessarily to represent serious pathology, with the possible exception of the oldest children in Factor III_3. In Factor IV_3, it would be more appropriate to talk about a general vulnerability; as already noted, such sensitivity to marginal stimulation may be a favorable prognostic sign (Smith, Sjöholm, and Nielzén, 1975). In contrast, when the most infantile and stimulus-deviant signs of projection are found in the middle and older age groups, as in Factor 5_3, they doubtlessly represent something more serious than mere oversensitivity to environmental factors.

We have assumed that signs of *discontinuous breaks* in either the MCT or AI test are more serious the more stabilized the subject's conception of reality should be (according to his cognitive level). Thus, a zero-phase in the MCT or a sudden shift from an adult AI to a primitive one would probably be signs of severe mental disorder in an adolescent but not in a 7-year-old. In Factor XII_1, the subjects have clearly discontinuous AI serials. Because the factor includes subjects age 7 to 13, however, it does not show a consistent profile of severe clinical symptoms. In Factor V_2, it is quite obvious that AI regressions do not necessarily constitute serious signs in young and cognitively immature subjects. With the systematic differentiation of younger and older subjects in conjunction with Factor 9_2, and when comparing this factor with Factor IV_2, it becomes quite clear that only in the upper half of our age range do signs of discontinuity clearly attest to psychotic or near-psychotic disturbances. The age difference in this correlation may have been enhanced by the fact that disturbances of this kind are clinically more difficult to identify in young children than in adolescents.

Among the most severe clinical symptoms are paroxysmal anxiety (in 12- to 16-year-olds), disturbed reality contact, near-psychotic reactions of other kinds, and feelings of impending disaster. We have just mentioned that these symptoms are likely to go together with signs of discontinuity in the tests, particularly as far as adolescents are concerned. As shown in Factor IV$_2$, open displays of fear and terror in the MCT are also common in these subjects. Instead of binding their anxiety in black perceptual structures as, for example, phobic patients would be likely to do, these subjects tend to bypass the possibilities offered by their perceptual world when expressing anxiety, and use more direct and primitive channels — not unlike immature 4- to 5-year-old normal children (see Chapter 3). A corollary to this is a lack of defensive capacity, which manifests itself in fusion between the hero and the threat in young children and inefficient or leaking mechanisms in older ones.

Factor I$_1$ brings up *the borderline issue.* We do not mean that these subjects demonstrate borderline pathology in a very typical way; two of the six subjects combined with another one to form a more seriously disturbed factor when process discontinuities were stressed in alternative 2. Clinical impressions of the majority of these subjects together with their permanent regressions in the AI test (incongruent with their ages) are, however, bound to arouse suspicions. According to Ross (1976), the central defect in the borderline person is "in the organizing structure of the self" (p. 308); at the same time, one sees "no break with reality, as in the psychotic . . . no avenue for escape" (p. 310). With our test instruments true psychotics at this adolescent age are likely to show discontinuous interruptions of reality testing, not permanent restriction to a more or less constant level of primitive functioning. The inability to integrate positive and negative introjects, which, according to Kernberg (1975), is typical of borderline patients, is revealed in children by the simultaneous coexistence of different organizations and, on the whole, by a primitive, unintegrated system of defenses (Ekstein and Wright, 1952). It is of particular interest to note the fantasies of space travel in these children since, in a way, the AI serials of our youngsters also seem to reflect a kind of distancing defense. Instead of acknowledging AIs as part of themselves, these adolescents identify the AIs with outside reality; the AIs become part of the projection screen and hence do not change in relative size as the projection distance becomes greater than the fixation distance. At the same time, the permanently primitive AIs of these adolescents are reminiscent of the dishabituation phenomena described by Nyman, Nyman, and Nylander (1978) as typical of nonregressive schizophrenia.

In Factor VI_1, we found a striking discrepancy between these adolescent subjects' mature AIs, reflecting *an adequate self-concept*, and their *immature way of evading* the MCT threat. Such discrepancies have been described by Anna Freud (1965) as typical of many disturbed children. It is interesting to learn that, according to her, parents often find these partial regressions very alarming; in our own factor description we pointed out that therapists often felt particularly worried about these children. However, the concern may be unfounded in these cases. According to Anna Freud, the partial regression often serves a progressive purpose. Langer (1969) notes that these children regress one step into a cul-de-sac in order to be able to take several steps forward along the main thoroughfare.

It is commonly agreed that *compulsive defenses* can be effective custodians, guarding against the breakthrough of primitive affect. Prepuberty seems to be an age where such defenses are particularly active even in normal children (see Blos, 1962). Referring to the frequency of compulsive signs in our own tests, we concluded in Chapter 2 that they appear to serve a preparatory purpose, anchoring these children securely in outside reality before the problems of puberty become dominant. In our analysis we find compulsive defenses among the much younger children clustered in Factor 9_1. The factor is undoubtedly small, but it leaves room for speculation about these advanced defenses' serving a temporary role as "regression inhibitors" even in children at early school age. What was most typical of the children in Factor 9_1 was their subsequent positive development. Just as in children on the verge of puberty, these children's compulsive defenses may have facilitated the extroverted activity which was probably instrumental in overcoming their depressive retardation (see also Factor X_2).

To conclude this discussion, we would like to find out whether our factor groupings illustrate the difference between structural and reactive childhood disorders (see Harrison and McDermott, 1972). Structural disorders reflect an imbalance of various functions *within* the person, while reactive disorders can be traced directly to environmental circumstances and are likely to recede when these circumstances are changed. If we maintain that borderline conditions reflect a central structural defect, they obviously belong to the group of structural disorders (Factor I_1). The prepsychotic or psychotic Factor IV_2 also belongs to this group. Factor III_1 may at first seem to belong to the reactive group because the neurotic concerns of these children appear to be direct reflections of their parental relations. These problems, however, have already become internalized to such an extent that environmental changes alone would not be likely to solve them.

Reactive disorders are better illustrated by Factor III_2 and to some extent by Factor XI_1, where there seems to be a direct relation between the child's depressive mood and a stressful home environment. Factor IV_3 also summarizes primarily reactive conditions. Here the increased vulnerability of the subjects renders even a fairly normal home environment potentially dangerous. These are the so-called difficult children. This last factor also makes it clear that the nature-nurture controversy is not necessarily involved in the distinction between structural and reactive disorders, but the distinction may be decisive for the choice of therapeutic intervention.

CONCLUSION

Our study used two process-oriented techniques to describe reactions of anxiety and strategies of defense in 72 normal schoolchildren (7–15 years of age), 55 normal preschool children (4–6 years of age), and 75 clinical children (4–16 years of age). All of the clinical children had anxiety in some form as a common denominator. A pilot group of 30 clinical children was also used to facilitate predictions for the larger clinical group. In order to obtain some information regarding the child's cognitive development, all children were given Piaget's landscape test of cognitive egocentrism. The larger clinical group was described with respect to a numer of symptoms and behavior characteristics believed to be pertinent to the main problem area under consideration.

Neither the afterimage (AI) test nor the meta-contrast technique (MCT) had been used before with children. The issue of reliability has therefore been a major concern (see the discussions in Chapters 2 and 3). An expected consequence of low reliability would be a more or less random distribution of data. Since the correlations discussed by us are quite high, the reliability of the data on which they are based is assumed to be at least acceptable. It could perhaps be argued that our correlations are random occurrences among a mass of possible associations. Results emanating from the various samples, however, support each other to a high, even very high, degree. Where direct cross-validation was not possible, new findings seem to fit within the framework of previous ones. In addition, some of the more expected findings attest to the general usefulness of our scoring methods and schemes of interpretation.

Both test methods rest on the model of percept genesis presented in the Introduction. Our general impression is of a reasonably good fit between this model and the analysis of our data in terms of a broader-reaching dynamic-developmental perspective. We admit that some loose ends remain and that some assumptions may have been too readily taken for granted. Our main excuse is the wealth of new information generated by our study; it has simply not been possible to develop the PG model sufficiently to let it alone account for all results. Instead, we have referred to related dynamic and cognitive theories. In doing so, we have tried to keep the door open for comparisons with a great number of investigations of normal and pathological child development. Too much isolation within a unique operational model would render such comparisons rather difficult.

The Descriptive Instruments

The MCT and the AI test have both served well as instruments for laying bare adaptive and defensive functioning in children. For the MCT, the lower age limit seems to be around 4 years (slightly lower for cognitively mature children). As far as the AI test is concerned, the limit is around 5 years (provided that the test is not simply used as an instrument to measure cognitive maturity). It is thus now possible to collect comparable data concerning PG processes and other aspects of adaptive and defensive functioning in young children as well as adolescents, mature adults, and elderly people. This ability to use the same instruments from early childhood to old age is rather unusual in the field of psychology.

That the MCT furnishes information regarding anxiety reactions and defensive strategies is known from previous research. What is new in our study is not only the introduction of younger age groups, but also of completely new scoring categories, such as primitive defenses on a behavioral level, leaking mechanisms, fusion between the hero and the threat, and retention of several alternative meanings simultaneously. When knowledge of these dimensions is brought to bear on adults, new insights into adaptive functioning may be gained, particularly in psychopathological groups of subjects. The consistent use of very primitive adaptive and defensive devices among many of the older clinical subjects in the present sample is one case in point. Another is the fluctuating regressive functioning typical of many people caught in unsolvable conflicts; when abrupt, these regressions may be psychotic in kind.

The AI test has been used to study anxiety in adults. It can also be used to study anxiety in children, even if the cognitive immaturity of young subjects may interfere with the results. Other useful dimensions pertain to hypersensitive reactions, process discontinuity, and degree of egocentrism. We also wish to point out the possibility of using the AI test for the detection of depressive tendencies. Although it does not differentiate between clinical and normal cases as clearly as the MCT, it seems to reflect a general tendency of retardation, which might be a basic characteristic of marginal as well as severe depressive reactions.

All through the present study it has been quite obvious that the scoring categories have to be adjusted to the age and cognitive maturity of the subjects. We shall refer below to the different manifestations of anxiety in different maturity groups. Other test signs that take on a different meaning with younger children are signs of discontinuity. Zero-phases in the MCT and regressions to primitive images in the AI test are indications of severe disturbances in children 12 to 16 years of age but are much less serious in young children who have not yet established their perceptual-cognitive frames of reference. The same is true of signs of open fright in the MCT situation, total disappearances of several AIs in a row, and many other signs.

It is important in PG testing to distinguish between late and early signs. Late signs supposedly indicate the present level of adaptation, while early signs belong to latent levels in the functional hierarchy. Hero duplication for instance, dominates late PG phases at early school age, but eventually disappears, although it may be found in early PG phases. The differentiation between early and late phases, however, is often difficult to make in preschool children, many of whom never report a stable C-phase. Here P-phases are very close to the C-phase, and new forms and meanings are continuously created at the

C-phase level under the immediate influence of the P-phases. This is one reason why many preschool children around the age of 5 normally and easily fill the world with their own subjective contents.

ANXIETY

We have adopted Schur's (1953, 1958) position that anxiety manifestations run from a pole of primary anxiety, where primitive discharge phenomena are most openly displayed, to one of much less intense and more affect-laden reactions to anticipated danger, reactions which would be unthinkable without a well-developed representational (inner) world. In between these poles, we find anxiety reactions that are still bound to the appearance or disappearance of a real, external object which represents danger to the subject.

A middle stage was first identified in the MCT protocols of some of the normal preschool children (Chapter 3). These children did not react to the threatening stimulus by reporting impressions of dark fields on the projection screen or similar signs associated with anxiety and apprehension in older children. Instead, they reacted directly by turning away from the screen, trying to walk out of the room, seeking shelter with the experimenter, reporting sudden somatic needs, etc. In other words, they displayed fright of something dangerous in their surroundings rather than unpleasant feelings inside themselves.

Internalized anxiety reactions were noted among the normal children, from preschool age upwards. Instead of outright fright, the negative affect was projected at the perceptual level. Undefended-against anxiety might in such cases be represented by black perceptual structures, broken structures, dissolution of existing defensive structures, and the like (see Chapter 8, in particular). As expected, these signs were more common among the anxiety-ridden clinical subjects than among the normals.

Primary anxiety was not represented in the normal group but appeared in the clinical group as paroxysmal anxiety. To be sure, in subjects with reported outbursts of paroxysmal anxiety, signs of open fright in the testing situation were often mixed with so-called severe signs of anxiety at the perceptual level. One obvious reason for this would be that these subjects did not regress all the way to primary anxiety reactions in the testing situation. If such regressions had occurred, the subjects would not have been able to complete the tests. Very young children with a high propensity for panic reactions were generally not testable.

Normally, direct reactions of fright were confined to a relatively early stage of cognitive development characterized by preoperational thinking, a fragmentary internal representation, and a still rather diffuse differentiation between self and nonself. Children at this stage, we reasoned, were not capable of internalizing their fright. As predicted, such overt reactions were still quite common at more advanced cognitive levels in the clinical group.

DEFENSIVE STRATEGIES

Defenses against noninternalized anxiety were expected to manifest themselves in overt reactions, seemingly directed against external danger rather than internal affects. (As was pointed out in Chapter 3, Freud himself saw specific motor responses in infants as possible precursors of adult defenses.) These direct reactions were expected to be marked by these children's egocentric thinking. We found children shutting their eyes or turning their heads away from the screen as if the threat would cease to exist the moment they could no longer see it. We equated this kind of defense with primitive or direct denial and classified it as transitory, or nonstructural.

In cognitively egocentric children with a more developed representational world, i.e., children in whom thought is no longer explicitly tied to action, we observed that the eye-shutting strategy was projected onto the boy in B_2. Instead of shutting his own eyes, the child was now able to let a stand-in for himself shut its eyes. This defensive stage is relatively brief and does not last beyond the very first school years. Traces of the hero's eye shutting can, however, be found at early PG stages in much older children. The childish defensive strategy obviously remains a *latent* possibility.

Concomitant with this change at early school age, we have also scored hero duplication. The narcissistic character of this defense seems particularly noteworthy—the threat is reduced to a nonthreatening self-reflection. As normal children grow older and become cognitively more mature, hero duplication no longer seems to serve so effectively. Hence older children may make the twin representing the threatening A_2 turn its head away. Such defensive strategies are typically adult and belong to the defense cluster of isolation. Like eye shutting, hero duplication may remain a latent possibility that appears early in the PG even after it has ceased to be effective.

Turning away the head of the threat foreshadows the period of prepuberty, a time of many compulsive reactions. In our normal 12- to 13-year-olds, the subjective side seemed effectively suppressed. We have assumed this emphasis on adaptation to external reality to be a preparation for the emotional turmoil and regressive reactions of puberty and adolescence, or, to use PG terminology, that it represents a consolidation of the final C-phase before the renewed reconstruction of early P-phase formations and the simultaneous emergence of new aspects of reality (see Chapter 2). In any case, the compulsive forms of defense (isolation, negation, intellectualization) are relatively late developments.

What has been termed "repression" in studies of adults—reports of a "decathected" bust or mask instead of a live A_2—cannot be traced very far back into childhood. Since psychoanalysts generally assume repression to be a defense against genital impulses, we expected to find these reports rather often among our youngest children. One reason for our failure to do so was pointed out in Chapter 3: the repressive defensive structures seen in adults would probably be as frightening to a young child as a living thing. Instead, we started to look for alternative signs of repression which would seem more harmless to the child. In this regard, we scored reports of a dismembered A_2 in several subjects. Yet these signs were still not as typical of the youngest subjects as we had anticipated. Perhaps repression is not quite such an early defensive strategy as many psychoanalysts have maintained.

One of the late strategies was isolation. In spite of its rarity at early school age, we were able to identify an analogous but much more primitive strategy among preschool children. What attracted our attention were the attempts of some small children to isolate physically the threatening A_2 from the boy in B_2, e.g., by using their hands to section off the area on the projection screen where A_2 had just appeared, or by employing various magic rituals in front of the screen. Even if we felt quite convinced that this behavior might very well be a precursor of adult isolation — it reminded us of Freud's speculation about flight with unaverted eyes as a prototype — we were at first slightly puzzled by the lack of continuity in time between this early form and the more common appearance of the adult forms at prepuberty. The observation of advanced compulsive defenses in a group of clinical children at early school age, however, convinced us that, if need be, full-fledged isolation could be effective long before prepuberty.

One of the most interesting strategies was projection. It peaked around the age of 5 and again at puberty. The young children saw extra animals and human beings in B (both series); the older children were more inclined to report slight changes in the appearance of B under the subliminal influence of A. While the flooding of percepts with subjective content thus appears to be a very common strategy in certain early stages of development, and is an adaptive rather than a defensive strategy, similar forms of projection must be considered clearly pathological when used by older children and adults. Projection may thus illustrate the very reasonable assumption that many adult defenses, even quite pathogenic forms, originate in perfectly innocuous devices used by the growing child to master the requirements of adaptation and growth.

Generally, as we have been able to show, the succession of defensive strategies over our age and cognitive maturity groups follows "field" observations rather closely. We started with direct denial among the immature 4- to 5-year-olds and ended up with compulsive mechanisms just before the age of puberty. However, possible precursors of late strategies could be identified relatively early. This also applies to depressive retardation, which we classify among the defensive countermeasures.

As we reported in Chapter 6, many clinicians feel uncertain about or even deny the existence of depression in children as young as ours, i.e., before or at early school age. According to our MCT and AI data, however, the reactions of joyless young children are quite similar in form to the reactions of depressed adults (although the narcissistic roots of depression are much more evident in the content of their reports). We thus concluded that depressive defenses relied on a very basic type of reaction to mental pain already discernible at early ontogenetic levels. What we call retardation here need not, naturally, be as pronounced as the symptoms typical of so-called endogenous depression.

As was the case with their anxiety reactions, the clinical children exhibited primitive defense mechanisms at relatively advanced age levels compared with normal children. A special study of possible factors behind this regressive functioning revealed that one prominent cause was probably the inefficiency of the more sophisticated mechanisms. Where anxiety "leaked through" these defensive barriers, the subject often went back to earlier forms of defense, even to such primitive denial as eye-shutting behavior. These early forms, as we noted in the case of eye shutting by the hero and hero duplication, must have remained as latent possibilities in the subject's defensive arsenal. The main problem, then, is why the child did not develop reasonably effective defenses with increasing age. Our data seem to indicate very early causes, far earlier than the age of 4 (the lower limit of our study).

A FINAL VIEW

As we have shown, our data clearly reflect a series of transitions in anxiety manifestations and defensive strategies from early preschool age to adolescence. This change is not arbitrary but reflects the progressive maturation of the child. The first major shift occurs around the age of 5 when the child's thought processes become less directly tied to action than before. The child is now able to internalize both anxiety reactions and the defensive measures taken to curb these reactions. Accordingly, the main defensive task is no longer to run away from external danger in fright, but to temper feelings of pain and discomfort, i.e., to master a danger which seems more and more to come from within rather than exclusively from without. As long as the cognitive perspective remains egocentric, the child's defensive strategy is closely linked to concrete impressions, or at least to their representations; by ignoring certain aspects of the world as the child understands it, he may be able to convince himself that they do not really exist. Not until these immediate appearances cease to dominate thought processes, at the second major point of transition a few years later, do the adult types of defense enter on the scene. At the same time anxiety becomes more a signal for anticipated inner danger.

The shift from a primarily external perspective to an internal one is often marked by exaggerated subjectivity (see Andersson, Johansson, Karlsson, and Ohlsson, 1972). As we have already discussed, children around 5 years of age are inclined to use projection in the MCT and, as it were, fill their conception of reality with new meaning from within. This stage apparently implies an important step toward forming the child's identity and could very well be called a first adolescence. Much later, after the compulsive period around the age of 12, the child enters a second adolescence, where growing subjectivity is often accompanied by signs of anxiety. Once again new perspectives on reality are created from within, although at a higher level of sophistication than at age 5 and with the use of more subtle projections. It is interesting to note that not only are these outbursts of subjectivity preceded by periods of one-sided reliance on outside reality or, if one likes, periods of consolidation, but also that the increased subjectivity is often accompanied by inhibiting measures reminiscent of those used by depressives. We thus venture the hypothesis that depressive retardation may be an exaggerated version of a normal reaction to mental discomfort (a rather common companion of subjective inflation).

The creation of new meaning from within occurs close to the C-phase level in children. In the PG theory this creation is covered by or akin to the concept of emergence (see the Introduction). Children are perfectly able to retain subjective contents and correct impressions side by side. The C-phase is not yet clearly separated from the P-phases. The two "adolescent" phases are particularly illuminating in this respect. One is reminded of Goethe's description of his own creative ventures as recurrent phases of adolescence. As mentioned earlier, we believe that creative activity in adulthood should, at least partly, be defined as reconstructive activity. In other words, the adult entertains reconstructed, previously dormant P-phase alternatives while, at the same time, his C-phase level remains distinct from this subjective activity. Naturally, reconstructed P-phase meanings may become so prominent and overwhelming in the adult's experiential world that he feels as if his youth or childhood had returned to him. A reconstruction of such proportions is likely, moreover, to be accompanied by feelings of anxiety—just as in adolescence.

It is important not to confuse states of subjective expansion in normal children with the more or less permanent regressions to primitive levels of functioning in clinical children suffering from anxiety. As is clearly demonstrated by our test methods, normal children play with their alternative interpretations and enjoy the ambiguities and contradictions created by them. Anxious children regress to a primitive level of functioning in order to avoid the problems inherent in these very contradictions; they prefer a simplified, more secure world of experience to a world on a level with their own age and cognitive maturity. Hence they are unable to make full use of their potential. One factor behind their tendency to regress seems to be their greater vulnerability, which, at least in part, grows out of the lack of defensive resources. In this situation, forms of defense such as isolation (i.e., the separation of perception and dangerous emotion from each other) may serve as a life preserver even for children at early school age. Such strategies probably protect the child from too permanent a fixation to primitive forms of defense or even from the danger of retreat into psychotic episodes.

Although our anxiety-ridden children did use primitive defenses more readily than normal children, it would be rash to consider all regressions—apart from the adaptive ones—as abnormal, with the negative connotations of that word. Occasional lapses into primitive defenses may be perfectly normal, as in extreme states of exhaustion or euphoria. Some normal people and some developmental phases are undoubtedly more prone to such lapses than others—and the clinical children and adolescents obviously even more so. As the PG processes of our children demonstrate, a person is likely to use primitive defenses as an alternative. These defenses often dominate P-phases close to the C-phase in young children, and they still tend to appear in the percept genesis of older children, but now in P-phases more remote from the C-phase. Hence, the full-fledged PG process can be seen to reflect the developmental stratification of the subject's experiential world.

The perspective on mental functioning supplied by our test data lends itself readily to combinations with dynamic theories of personality, in general, and psychoanalytic ones, in particular. Generally, the substance of our findings agrees with clinical observations although it differs from such observations on a number of important points. In addition, our data present several advantages. As reconstructions of preconscious material at the perceptual level, they offer both more basic information regarding mental functioning than most conventional test studies and more reliable information than the usual clinical case descriptions, at least descriptions based on childhood recollections of adult patients. Another benefit of our experimental approach is that it makes possible a systematic combination of observations from both clinical children and normal ones and that these observations can be appraised against the background of longitudinal studies of adults. Only as part of a broad spectrum of human development do the characteristics of anxiety-ridden children like ours really become comprehensible.

If our instruments are used as descriptive-diagnostic tools, they may provide the practicing clinician with hypotheses that further his therapeutic endeavors. Let us give a few simplified examples. It is always important to know at what developmental level the patient's anxiety is likely to manifest itself and also whether it will remain latent or begin to appear openly. Similarly, the PG methods—and the MCT in particular—can inform us about the maturity of the patient's defensive strategy, disclosing traces of primitiveness or narcissism, and can tell us about the breadth and firmness of the defensive repertoire. This kind of knowledge is imperative even if, in these age groups, a therapist is mostly bound to the use of supportive therapeutic measures. Without a thorough knowledge of the child's defensive functioning, the therapist cannot know what resources to cultivate in order to promote adaptation, when to tread particularly carefully so as not to risk a psychotic break, when to hold the child rather severely in check and when to give free rein. For instance, if severe anxiety is shielded by depressive retardation or compulsive isolation, the treatment plan should be different from cases with less severe anxiety behind the defensive armor. Every skilled clinician eventually learns these things in the course of treating the patient. Good test instruments may, however, inform or at least caution him from the very beginning of his therapeutic work. The concrete form and systematic developmental order in which data are presented in PG tests make them particularly suited for such a use, at least when the therapy is informed by a dynamic theory.

This use of the PG method in clinical settings should not conceal its possible application in more normal problem areas. The description of child development offered by our instruments may serve as a background to more general discussions about the treatment and education of children, about how best to support their creative leanings, and about how to balance their attempts to build their own identity with socialization forces. These are far-reaching questions; the data generated here highlight a humble beginning toward answering them.

REFERENCES

Abraham, K. (1911), Notes on the Psycho-Analytical Investigation and Treatment of Manic-Depressive Insanity and Allied Conditions. In: *Selected Papers on Psychoanalysis.* London: Hogarth Press, 1927, pp. 137-156.

Almgren, P.-E. (1971), Relations between Perceptual Defenses, Defined by the Meta-Contrast Technique and Adaptive Patterns in Two Serial Behavior Tests. *Psychological Research Bulletin, Lund University,* 11 (3).

Andersson, A. L.; Fries, I.; & Smith, G. J. W. (1970), Change in Afterimage and Spiral Aftereffect Serials due to Anxiety Caused by Subliminal Threat. *Scandinavian Journal of Psychology,* 11:7-16.

_____ Johansson, A.; Karlsson, B; & Ohlsson, M. (1972), On Self-Nonself Interaction in Early Childhood as Revealed by the Spiral Aftereffect Duration. In: *Visual Aftereffects and the Individual as an Adaptive System,* ed. A. L. Andersson, Å. Nilsson, E. Ruuth, & G. J. W. Smith. Lund: Gleerup, pp. 199-208.

_____ Nilsson, Å.; & Henriksson, N. G. (1970), Personality Differences between Accident-Loaded and Accident-Free Young Car Drivers. *British Journal of Psychology,* 61:409-421.

_____ _____ Ruuth, E.; & Smith, G. J. W. (1972), *Visual Aftereffects and the Individual as an Adaptive System.* Lund: Gleerup.

_____ & Weikert, C. (1974), Adult Defensive Organization as Related to Adaptive Regulation of Spiral Aftereffect Duration. *Social Behavior & Personality,* 2:56-75.

Anthony, E. J. (1975a), Childhood Depression. In: *Depression and Human Existence,* ed. E. J. Anthony & T. Benedek. Boston: Little, Brown, pp. 231-273.

_____ (1975b), The Juvenile and Preadolescent Periods of the Human Life Cycle. In: *American Handbook of Psychiatry,* Vol. 1. New York: Basic Books, pp. 368-381.

_____ (1975c), Neurotic Disorders. In: *Comprehensive Textbook of Psychiatry,* Vol. 2, ed. A. M. Freedman, H. I. Kaplan, & B. J. Sadock. Baltimore: Williams & Wilkins, pp. 2143-2160.

Bibring, E. (1953), The Mechanism of Depression. In: *Affective Disorders,* ed. P.

195

Greenacre. New York: International Universities Press, pp. 13-48.

Bibring, G. L.; Dwyer, T. F.; Huntington, D. S.; et al. (1961), A Study of the Psychological Process in Pregnancy and of the Earliest Mother-Child Relationship, II: Methodological Considerations. *The Psychoanalytic Study of the Child,* 16:25-72. New York: International Universities Press.

Blos, P. (1962), *On Adolescence: A Psychoanalytic Interpretation.* New York: Free Press.

Bowlby, J. (1973), *Attachment and Loss, II: Separation, Anxiety and Anger.* London: Hogarth Press.

Cameron, N. (1963), *Personality Development and Psychopathology: A Dynamic Approach.* Boston: Houghton Mifflin.

Cheatam, P. G. (1952), Visual Perceptual Latency as a Function of Stimulus Brightness and Contour Shape. *Journal of Experimental Psychology,* 43:369-380.

Eberhard, G.; Johnson, G.; Nilsson, L.; & Smith, G. J. W. (1965), Clinical and Experimental Approaches to the Description of Depression and Antidepressive Therapy. *Acta Psychiatrica Scandinavica,* 41 (Suppl. 186).

Edgcumbe, R., & Burgner, M. (1972), Some Problems in the Conceptualization of Early Object Relationships, I. *The Psychoanalytic Study of the Child,* 27:283-314. New York: Quadrangle.

Eissler, K. R. (1959), On Isolation. *The Psychoanalytic Study of the Child,* 14:29-60. New York: International Universities Press.

Elkind, D. (1967), Egocentrism in Adolescence, *Child Development,* 38: 1025-1034.

Ekstein, R., & Wright, D. G. (1952), The Space Child. *Bulletin of the Menninger Clinic,* 16:211-224.

Engel, G., & Schmale, A. (1972), Conservation-Withdrawal: A Primary Regulatory Process for Organic Homeostasis. In: *Physiology, Emotion and Psychosomatic Illness* (Ciba Foundation Symposium 8). Amsterdam: Elsevier.

Fenichel, O. (1945), *The Psychoanalytic Theory of Neurosis.* London: Routledge & Kegan Paul.

Fraiberg, S. (1977), *Insights from the Blind.* New York: Basic Books.

Freud, A. (1936), *The Ego and the Mechanisms of Defense. The Writings of Anna Freud,* 2. New York: International Universities Press, 1966.

———— (1965), *Normality and Pathology in Childhood. The Writings of Anna Freud,* 6. New York: International Universities Press.

———— (1970), The Symptomatology of Childhood: A Preliminary Attempt at Classification. *The Psychoanalytic Study of the Child,* 25:19-41. New York: International Universities Press.

Freud, S. (1915), Instincts and Their Vicissitudes. *Standard Edition,* 14:117-140. London: Hogarth Press, 1957.

———— (1920), Beyond the Pleasure Principle. *Standard Edition,* 18:3-64. London: Hogarth Press, 1955.

———— (1926), Inhibitions, Symptoms and Anxiety. *Standard Edition,* 20:77-175. London: Hogarth Press, 1959.

Fries, I., & Smith, G. J. W. (1970), Influence of Physiognomic Stimulus Properties on Afterimage Adaptation. *Perceptual & Motor Skills,* 31:267-271.

Gardner, R. W.; Jackson, D. N.; & Messick, S. J. (1960), *Personality Organization in Cognitive Controls and Intellectual Abilities* [*Psychological Issues,* Monogr. 8]. New York: International Universities Press.

Gedo, J. E., & Goldberg, A. (1973), *Models of the Mind: A Psychoanalytic Theory.* Chicago: University of Chicago Press.

Greenacre, P. (1967), The Influence of Infantile Trauma on Genetic Patterns. In:

Psychic Trauma, ed. S. S. Furst. New York: Basic Books, pp. 108-153.

Greenspan, S. I. (1980), *Intelligence and Adaptation: An Integration of Psychoanalytic and Piagetian Developmental Psychology* [*Psychological Issues,* Monogr. 47/48]. New York: International Universities Press.

Hagberg, B. (1973), A Prospective Study of Patients in Chronic Hemodialysis, III. *Journal of Psychosomatic Research,* 18:151-160.

Hartmann, H. (1939), *Ego Psychology and the Problem of Adaptation.* New York: International Universities Press, 1958.

Harrison, S. I., & McDermott, J. F., Eds. (1972), *Childhood Psychopathology.* New York: International Universities Press.

Holley, J. W., & Guilford, J. P. (1964), A Note on the G Index of Agreement. *Educational & Psychological Measurement,* 24:749-753.

_____ & Risberg, J. (1972), On the D Estimate of Discriminatory Effectiveness. *Psychological Research Bulletin, Lund University,* 12 (12).

_____ & Nilsson, I. K. (1973), On the Validity of Some Clinical Measures. *Psychological Research Bulletin, Lund University,* 13 (4).

Holzman, P. S., & Klein, G. S. (1954), Cognitive System-Principles of Levelling and Sharpening: Individual Differences in Assimilation Effects of Visual Time-Error. *Journal of Psychology,* 37:105-122.

Jacobson, E. (1957), Denial and Repression. *Journal of the American Psychoanalytic Association,* 5:61-92.

Jaensch, E. R., et al. (1929), *Grundformen menschlichen Seins.* Berlin: Elsner.

_____ et al. (1930), *Studie zur Psychologie menschlicher Typen.* Leipzig: Barth.

Kernberg, O. (1975), *Borderline Conditions and Pathological Narcissism.* New York: Aronson.

Klein, G. S., & Schlesinger, H. J. (1949), Where Is the Perceiver in Perceptual Theory? *Journal of Personality,* 18:32-47.

_____ Spence, D.; Holt, R. R.; & Gourevitch, S. (1958), Cognition without Awareness: Subliminal Influences upon Conscious Thought. *Journal of Abnormal & Social Psychology,* 59:167-176.

Kolb, L. C. (1968), *Noyes' Modern Clinical Psychiatry.* Philadelphia: Saunders.

Kragh, U. (1955), *The Actual-Genetic Model of Perception-Personality.* Lund: Gleerup.

_____ (1969), *DMT-Defense Mechanism Test.* Stockholm: Skandinaviska Testförlaget.

_____ & Smith, G. J. W. (1970), *Percept-Genetic Analysis.* Lund: Gleerup.

_____ _____ (1974), Forming New Patterns of Experience: A Classical Problem Viewed within a Percept-Genetic Model. *Psychological Research Bulletin, Lund University,* 14 (6).

Kroh, O. (1922), *Subjektive Anschauungsbilder bei Jugendlichen.* Göttingen: Vandenhoeck & Ruprecht.

Langer, J. (1969), *Theories of Development.* New York: Holt.

Lehmann, H. E. (1959), Psychiatric Concepts of Depression: Nomenclature and Classification. *Canadian Psychiatric Association Journal,* 4 (Suppl. 1-2).

Lindbom, K. (1968), Perceptual Defense Mechanisms Registered by the Meta-Contrast Technique in Normal and Pathologic Children. *Scandinavian Journal of Psychology,* 9:109-116.

Magnusson, P.-A.; Nilsson, Å.; & Henriksson, N. G. (1977), Psychogenic Vertigo within an Anxiety Frame of Reference: An Experimental Study. *British Journal of Medical Psychology,* 50:187-201.

Mahler, M. S. (1961), On Sadness and Grief in Infancy and Childhood: Loss and

Restoration of the Symbiotic Love Object. *The Psychoanalytic Study of the Child,* 16:332-351. New York: International Universities Press.

Malmquist, C. P. (1972), Depressions in Childhood and Adolescence. In: *Annual Progress in Child Psychiatry and Child Development,* ed. S. Chess & A. Thomas. New York: Brunner/Mazel, pp. 507-535.

Mendelson, M. (1974), *Psychoanalytic Concepts of Depression,* 2nd Ed. New York: Spectrum.

Nilsson, Å., & Almgren, P.-E. (1970), Para-Natal Emotional Adjustment: A Prospective Investigation of 165 Women. Part II: The Influence of Background Factors, Psychiatric History, Parental Relations, and Personality Characteristics. *Acta Psychiatrica Scandinavica,* Suppl. 220:63-141.

Nilsson, I. K. & Larsson, K. (1972), En Q-faktoranalytisk studie över testpsykologiska skillnader mellan en grupp schizofrena patienter och en normalgrupp. Master's thesis, Department of Psychology, Lund University.

Novick, J., & Kelly, K. (1970), Projection and Externalization. *The Psychoanalytic Study of the Child,* 25:69-95. New York: International Universities Press.

Nyman, G. E. (1975), The Clinical Picture of Non-Regressive Schizophrenia. *Nordisk Psykiatrisk Tidskrift,* 29:249-258.

———— Nyman, A. K.; & Nylander, B. I. (1978), Non-Regressive Schizophrenia, I: A Comparative Study of Clinical Picture, Social Prognosis, and Heredity. *Acta Psychiatrica Scandinavica,* 57:165-192.

Palmquist, A. (1974), Jämförelser av DMT och MCT baserade på fyra kliniska grupper. Doctoral thesis, Department of Psychology, Lund University.

Piaget, J. (1926), *The Child's Conception of the World.* London: Kegan Paul, 1929.

———— (1947), *The Psychology of Intelligence.* London: Routledge & Kegan Paul, 1950.

———— (1923), *The Language and Thought of the Child.* New York: Meridan, 1955.

———— & Inhelder, B. (1941), *Le developpement des quantités chez l'enfant.* Neuchatel: Delachaux & Niestlé.

———— ———— (1948), *The Child's Conception of Space.* London: Routledge & Kegan Paul, 1956.

———— ———— (1966), *The Psychology of the Child.* New York: Basic Books, 1969.

Rie, H. E. (1966), Depression in Childhood: A Survey of Some Pertinent Contributions. *Journal of the American Academy of Child Psychiatry,* 5:653-685.

Ross, M. (1976), The Borderline Diathesis. *International Review of Psycho-Analysis,* 3:305-321.

Ruuth, E. (1970), Afterimage Perception and Size-Distance Judgment in Preschool Children. *Psychological Research Bulletin, Lund University,* 10 (4).

———— & Andersson, A. L. (1971), Emmert's Law Reconsidered: A Developmental Study of Visual Afterimages. *Psychological Research Bulletin, Lund University,* 11 (8).

———— & Smith, G. J. W. (1969), Projected Afterimages and Cognitive Maturity. *Scandinavian Journal of Psychology,* 10:209-214.

Sander, F. (1928), Experimentelle Ergebnisse der Gestaltpsychologie. *Berichte über den X Kongress der experimentellen Psychologie in Bonn 1927,* pp. 23-28.

Sandler, A. M. (1975), The Significance of Piaget's Work for Psychoanalysis. Presented as Anna Freud Memorial Lecture in Psychoanalysis, University College, London.

Sandler, J., & Joffe, W. G. (1965), Notes on Childhood Depression. *International*

Journal of Psycho-Analysis, 46:88-96.

_____ _____ (1968), Psychoanalytic Psychology and Learning Theory. In: *The Role of Learning in Psychotherapy,* ed. R. Porter. London: Churchill, pp. 274-287.

_____ & Rosenblatt, B. (1962), The Concept of the Representational World. *The Psychoanalytic Study of the Child,* 17:128-145. New York: International Universities Press.

Schulterbrandt, J. G., & Raskin, A., Eds. (1977), *Depression in Childhood: Diagnosis, Treatment, and Conceptual Models.* New York: Raven Press.

Schur, M. (1953), The Ego in Anxiety. In: *Drives, Affects, Behavior,* ed. R. M. Loewenstein. New York: International Universities Press, pp. 67-103.

_____ (1958), The Ego and the Id in Anxiety. *The Psychoanalytic Study of the Child,* 13:190-220. New York: International Universities Press.

Sjöbäck, H. (1973), *The Psychoanalytic Theory of Defensive Processes.* Lund: Gleerup.

Smedslund, J. (1967), *Psykologi.* Oslo: Universitetsförlaget.

Smith, G. J. W. (1949), *Psychological Studies in Twin Differences.* Lund: Gleerup.

_____ (1975), MCT-metakontrasttekniken, interimrapport 1974-75. Lund: Department of Psychology (mimeo).

_____ & Carlsson, I. (1980), Can Preschool Children Be Creative? An Experimental Study with 4-6-Year-Olds. *Psychological Research Bulletin, Lund University,* 20 (7-8).

_____ Fries, I.; Andersson, A. L.; & Ried, J. (1971), Diagnostic Exploitation of Visual Aftereffect Measures in a Moderately Depressive Patient Group. *Scandinavian Journal of Psychology,* 12:67-79.

_____ & Henriksson, M. (1955), The Effect on an Established Percept of a Perceptual Process Beyond Awareness. *Acta Psychologica,* 11:346-355.

_____ _____ (1956), Studies in the Development of a Percept within Various Contexts of Perceived Reality. *Acta Psychologica,* 12:263-281.

_____ Johnson, G.; Ljunghill-Andersson, J.; & Almgren, P. E. (1970), *MCT-Meta kontrasttekniken.* Stockholm: Skandinaviska Testförlaget.

_____ & Klein, G. S. (1953), Cognitive Controls in Serial Behavior Patterns. *Journal of Personality,* 22:188-213.

_____ & Kragh, U. (1967), A Serial Afterimage Experiment in Clinical Diagnostics. *Scandinavian Journal of Psychology,* 8:52-64.

_____ _____ (1975), Creativity in Mature and Old Age. *Psychological Research Bulletin, Lund University,* 15 (7).

_____ _____ Eberhard, G.; & Johnson, G. (1970), Forms of Depression as Reflected in Negative Afterimage Serials. *Acta Psychiatrica Scandinavica,* 46 (Suppl. 219): 216-223.

_____ Ruuth, E.; Franzén, G.; & Sjöholm, L. (1972), Intermittent Regressions in a Serial Afterimage Experiment as Signs of Schizophrenia. *Scandinavian Journal of Psychology,* 13:27-33.

_____ & Sjöholm, L. (1970), Projected Afterimages after Manipulation of Cognitive Schemes in Children. *Scandinavian Journal of Psychology,* 11:274-279.

_____ _____ (1971), Afterimage Change in Children Following Reversal of Experimenter's Theoretical Message. *Perceptual & Motor Skills,* 32:899-904.

_____ _____ (1972), Autonomy of Visual Afterimages as Tested by Changing Projection Surface. *Perceptual & Motor Skills,* 35:539-547.

_____ _____ (1974a), Can Our Theory of Reality Influence Our Perception of

It? *Psychological Research Bulletin, Lund University,* 14 (1).

———— ———— (1974b), The Effect on His Visual Afterimages of a Subject's Defensive System in Interaction with the Afterimage Theory Presented to Him. *Scandinavian Journal of Psychology,* 15:255-262.

———— ———— & Nielzén, S. (1974), Sensitive Reactions and Afterimage Variegation. *Journal of Personality Assessment,* 38:41-47.

———— ———— ———— (1975), Individual Factors Affecting the Improvement of Anxiety during a Therapeutic Period of 1½ to 2 years. *Acta Psychiatrica Scandinavica,* 52:7-22.

———— ———— ———— (1976), Anxiety and Defense against Anxiety as Reflected in Percept-Genetic Formations. *Journal of Personality Assessment,* 40:151-161.

———— Spence, D. P., & Klein, G. S. (1959), Subliminal Effects of Verbal Stimuli. *Journal of Abnormal and Social Psychology,* 59:167-176.

———— & Westerlundh, B. (1980), Percept Genesis: A Process Perspective on Perception-Personality. In: *Review of Personality and Social Psychology,* Vol. 1, ed. L. Wheeler. Beverly Hills, Cal.: Sage Publications, pp. 94-124.

Spitz, R. A. (1961), Some Early Prototypes of Ego Defenses. *Journal of the American Psychoanalytic Association,* 9:626-651.

Symonds, P. M. (1945), *Defenses: The Dynamics of Human Adjustment.* New York: Appleton-Century-Crofts.

Tanner, J. M. (1971), Sequence, Tempo, and Individual Variation in the Growth and Development of Boys and Girls Aged 12 to 16. In: *New Directions in Childhood Psychopathology,* ed. S. I. Harrison & J. F. McDermott. New York: International Universities Press, 1980, pp. 182-202.

Vaillant, G. E. (1971), Theoretical Hierarchy of Adaptive Ego Mechanisms. *Archives of General Psychiatry,* 24:107-118.

Vujić, V., & Levi, K. (1939), *Die Pathologie der optischen Nachbilder und ihre klinische Verwertung.* Basel: Karger.

Werner, H. (1940), Studies on Contour: I. Qualitative Analyses. *American Journal of Psychology,* 47:40-64.

———— (1948), *Comparative Psychology of Mental Development,* (Rev. Ed.). New York: International Universities Press.

———— (1957), The Concept of Development from a Comparative and Organismic Point of View. In: *The Concept of Development,* ed D. B. Harris. Minneapolis: University of Minnesota Press, pp. 125-148.

Winnicott, D. W. (1953), Transitional Objects and Transitional Phenomena. *International Journal of Psycho-Analysis,* 34:89-97.

INDEX

ABOUT THE AUTHORS

GUDMUND J. W. SMITH received his Ph.D. from Lund University, Sweden, in 1949, and did his post-doctoral work at Harvard University from 1951 to 1953. Since 1960 he has been Professor and Head of the Doctoral Program in the Department of Psychology at Lund University. From 1955 to 1956 he was a Research Professor at the Research Center for Mental Health, New York University, and from 1957 to 1960 a Research Professor for the Swedish Council for Medical Research. He has also served as President of the Scandinavian Society of Scientific Psychology and was recently elected to the executive committee of the International Society for the Study of Behavioral Development. Dr. Smith is both author and co-author of numerous books and articles, many of which focus on the percept-genetic approach.

ANNA K. DANIELSSON received her M.A. from Lund University and is currently completing her Ph.D. work there. She received her psychoanalytic training in Copenhagen and is a member of the Danish Psychoanalytic Society. She has also studied at Zurich University and at the Hampstead Child Guidance Clinic in London. Between 1974 and 1979 she worked with Dr. Smith, and they have co-authored a number of publications related to the research presented in this monograph.

PSYCHOLOGICAL ISSUES

PSYCHOLOGICAL ISSUES

HERBERT J. SCHLESINGER, *Editor*

Editorial Board